TESTING
TREATMENTS

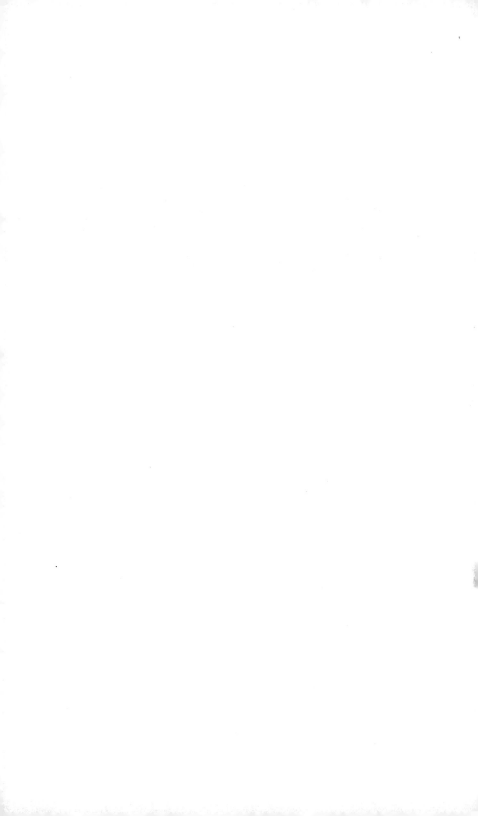

TESTING TREATMENTS

BETTER RESEARCH FOR BETTER HEALTHCARE

SECOND EDITION

**Imogen Evans, Hazel Thornton,
Iain Chalmers and Paul Glasziou**

Foreword Ben Goldacre

We dedicate this book to William Silverman (1917–2004),
who encouraged us repeatedly to challenge authority.

Testing Treatments
Better Research for Better Healthcare

First published in 2006 by The British Library
This second edition first published 2011 by Pinter & Martin Ltd

British Library Cataloguing in Publication Data
A catalogue record for this book is available from the British Library

ISBN 978-1-905177-48-6

Printed and bound in the EU by Hussar Books

This book has been printed on paper that is sourced and harvested from
sustainable forests and is FSC accredited

Pinter & Martin Ltd
6 Effra Parade
London SW2 1PS

www.pinterandmartin.com

Contents

About the authors

Imogen Evans practised and lectured in medicine in Canada and the UK before turning to medical journalism at *The Lancet*. From 1996 to 2005 she worked for the Medical Research Council, latterly in research ethics, and has represented the UK government on the Council of Europe Biomedical Ethics Committee.

Hazel Thornton, after undergoing routine mammography, was invited to join a clinical trial, but the inadequate patient information led to her refusal. However, it also encouraged her advocacy for public involvement in research to achieve outcomes relevant to patients. She has written and spoken extensively on this topic.

Iain Chalmers practised medicine in the UK and Palestine before becoming a health services researcher and directing the National Perinatal Epidemiology Unit and then the UK Cochrane Centre. Since 2003 he has coordinated the James Lind Initiative, promoting better controlled trials for better healthcare, particularly through greater public involvement.

Paul Glasziou is both a medical researcher and part-time General Practitioner. As a consequence of observing the gap between these, he has focused his work on identifying and removing the barriers to using high-quality research in everyday clinical practice. He was editor of the BMJ's *Journal of Evidence-Based Medicine*, and Director of the Centre for Evidence-Based Medicine in Oxford from 2003 to 2010. He is the author of several other books related to evidence-based practice. He is currently the recipient of a National Health and Medical Research Council Australia Fellowship which he commenced at Bond University in July, 2010.

Acknowledgements

We thank the following people for their valuable comments and other contributions that have helped us to develop the second edition of *Testing Treatments*:

Claire Allen, Doug Altman, Patricia Atkinson, Alexandra Barratt, Paul Barrow, Ben Bauer, Michael Baum, Sarah Boseley, Joan Box, Anne Brice, Rebecca Brice, Amanda Burls, Hamish Chalmers, Jan Chalmers, Yao-long Chen, Olivia Clarke, Catrin Comeau, Rhiannon Comeau, Katherine Cowan, John Critchlow, Sally Crowe, Philipp Dahm, Chris Del Mar, Jenny Doust, Mary Dixon-Woods, Ben Djulbegovic, Iain Donaldson, George Ebers, Diana Elbourne, Murray Enkin, Chrissy Erueti, Curt Furberg, Mark Fenton, Lester Firkins, Peter Gøtzsche, Muir Gray, Sally Green, Susan Green, Ben Goldacre, Metin Gülmezoğlu, Andrew Herxheimer, Jini Hetherington, Julian Higgins, Jenny Hirst, Jeremy Howick, Les Irwig, Ray Jobling, Bethan Jones, Karsten Juhl Jørgensen, Bridget Kenner, Debbie Kennett, Gill Lever, Alessandro Liberati, Howard Mann, Tom Marshall, Robert Matthews, Margaret McCartney, Dominic McDonald, Scott Metcalfe, Iain Milne, Martin McKee, Sarah Moore, Daniel Nicolae, Andy Oxman, Kay Pattison, Angela Raffle, June Raine, Jake Ranson, James Read, Kiley Richmond, Ian Roberts, Nick Ross, Peter Rothwell, Karen Sandler, Emily Savage-Smith, Marion Savage-Smith, John Scadding, Lisa Schwartz, Haleema Shakur, Ruth Silverman, Ann Southwell, Pete Spain, Mark Starr, Melissa Sweet, Tilli Tansey, Tom Treasure, Ulrich Tröhler, Liz Trotman, Liz Wager, Renee Watson, James Watt, Hywel Williams, Norman Williams, Steven Woloshin, Eleanor Woods, and Ke-hu Yang.

Iain Chalmers and Paul Glasziou are grateful to the National Institute for Health Research (UK) for support. Paul Glasziou is also grateful to the National Health and Medical Research Council (Australia).

And a special thank you to our publisher, Martin Wagner, of Pinter & Martin for his forbearance, cheerful encouragement, and cool head at all times.

Foreword

Medicine shouldn't be about authority, and the most important question anyone can ask on any claim is simple: 'how do you know?' This book is about the answer to that question.

There has been a huge shift in the way that people who work in medicine relate to patients. In the distant past, 'communications skills training', such as it was, consisted of how not to tell your patient they were dying of cancer. Today we teach students – and this is a direct quote from the hand-outs – how to 'work collaboratively with the patient towards an optimum health outcome'. Today, if they wish, at medicine's best, patients are involved in discussing and choosing their own treatments.

For this to happen, it's vital that everyone understands how we know if a treatment works, how we know if it has harms, and how we weigh benefits against harms to determine the risk. Sadly doctors can fall short on this, as much as anybody else. Even more sadly, there is a vast army out there, queuing up to mislead us.

First and foremost in this gallery of rogues, we can mislead ourselves. Most diseases have a natural history, getting better and worse in cycles, or at random: because of this, anything you do, if you act when symptoms are at their worst, might make a treatment seem to be effective, because you were going to get better anyway.

The placebo effect, similarly, can mislead us all: people really can get better, in some cases, simply from taking a dummy pill with no active ingredients, and by believing their treatments to be effective. As Robert M Pirsig said, in *Zen and the Art of Motorcycle Maintenance*: 'the real purpose of the scientific method is to make sure nature hasn't misled you into thinking you know something you actually don't know'.

But then there are the people who brandish scientific studies. If there is one key message from this book – and it is a phrase I have borrowed and used endlessly myself – it is the concept of a 'fair test'. Not all trials are born the same, because there are so many ways that a piece of scientific research can be biased, and erroneously give what someone, somewhere thinks should be the 'right' answer.

Sometimes evidence can be distorted through absent-mindedness, or the purest of motives (for all that motive should matter). Doctors, patients, professors, nurses, occupational therapists, and managers can all become wedded to the idea that one true treatment, in which they have invested so much personal energy, is golden.

Sometimes evidence can be distorted for other reasons. It would be wrong to fall into shallow conspiracy theories about the pharmaceutical industry: they have brought huge, lifesaving advances. But there is a lot of money at stake in some research, and for reasons you will see in this book, 90% of trials are conducted by industry. This can be a problem, when studies funded by industry are four times more likely to have a positive result for the sponsor's drug than independently funded trials. It costs up to $800m to bring a new drug to market: most of that is spent before the drug comes to market, and if the drug turns out to be no good, the money is already spent. Where the stakes are so high, sometimes the ideals of a fair test can fail.[1]

Equally, the way that evidence is communicated can be distorted, and misleading. Sometimes this can be in the presentation of facts and figures, telling only part of the story, glossing over flaws, and 'cherry picking' the scientific evidence which shows one treatment in a particular light.

But in popular culture, there can be more interesting processes at play. We have an understandable desire for miracle cures, even though research is frequently about modest improvements, shavings of risk, and close judgement calls. In the media, all too often this can be thrown aside in a barrage of words like 'cure', 'miracle', 'hope', 'breakthrough', and 'victim'.[2]

At a time when so many are so keen to take control of their own lives, and be involved in decisions about their own healthcare, it is sad to see so much distorted information, as it can only disempower. Sometimes these distortions are around a specific drug: the presentation in the UK media of Herceptin as a miracle cure for breast cancer is perhaps the most compelling recent example.[3]

Sometimes, though, in promoting their own treatments, and challenging the evidence against them, zealots and their friends in the media can do even greater damage, by actively undermining the public's very understanding of how we know if something is good for us, or bad for us.

Homoeopathy sugar pills perform no better than dummy sugar pills when compared by the most fair tests. But when confronted with this evidence, homoeopaths argue that there is something wrong with the whole notion of doing a trial, that there is some complicated reason why their pills, uniquely among pills, cannot be tested. Politicians, when confronted with evidence that their favoured teaching programme for preventing teenage pregnancy has failed, may fall into the same kind of special pleading. In reality, as this book will show, any claim made about an intervention having an effect can be subjected to a transparent fair test.[4]

Sometimes these distortions can go even deeper into undermining the public's understanding. A recent 'systematic review' of all the most fair and unbiased tests showed there was no evidence that taking antioxidant vitamin pills can prolong life (in fact, they may even shorten it). With this kind of summary – as explained beautifully in this book – clear rules are followed, describing where to look for evidence, what evidence can be included, and how its quality should be assessed. But when systematic reviews produce a result that challenges the claims of antioxidant supplement pill companies, newspapers and magazines are filled with false criticisms, arguing that individual studies for the systematic review have been selectively 'cherry picked', for reasons of political allegiance or frank corruption, that favourable evidence has been deliberately ignored, and so on.[5]

This is unfortunate. The notion of systematic review – looking at the totality of evidence – is quietly one of the most important innovations in medicine over the past 30 years. In defending their small corner of retail business, by undermining the public's access to these ideas, journalists and pill companies can do us all a great disservice.

And that is the rub. There are many reasons to read this book. At the simplest level, it will help you make your own decisions about your own health in a much more informed way. If you work in medicine, the chapters that follow will probably stand head and shoulders above any teaching you had in evidence-based medicine. At the population level, if more people understand how to make fair comparisons, and see whether one intervention is better than another, then as the authors argue, instead of sometimes fearing research, the public might actively campaign to be more involved in reducing uncertainties about the treatments that matter to them.

But there is one final reason to read this book, to learn the tricks of our trade, and that reason has nothing to do with practicality: the plain fact is, this stuff is interesting, and beautiful, and clever. And in this book it's explained better than anywhere else I've ever seen, because of the experience, knowledge, and empathy of the people who wrote it.

Testing Treatments brings a human focus to real world questions. Medicine is about human suffering, and death, but also human frailty in decision makers and researchers: and this is captured here, in the personal stories and doubts of researchers, their motivations, concerns, and their shifts of opinion. It's rare for this side of science to be made accessible to the public, and the authors move freely, from serious academic papers to the more ephemeral corners of medical literature, finding unguarded pearls from the discussion threads beneath academic papers, commentaries, autobiographies, and casual asides.

This book should be in every school, and every medical waiting room. Until then, it's in your hands. Read on.

Ben Goldacre
August 2011

Foreword to the first edition

This book is good for our health. It shines light on the mysteries of how life and death decisions are made. It shows how those judgements are often badly flawed and it sets a challenge for doctors across the globe to mend their ways.

Yet it accomplishes this without unnecessary scares; and it warmly admires much of what modern medicine has achieved. Its ambitions are always to improve medical practice, not disparage it.

My own first insight into entrenched sloppiness in medicine came in the 1980s when I was invited to be a lay member of a consensus panel set up to judge best practice in the treatment of breast cancer. I was shocked (and you may be too when you read more about this issue in Chapter 2 [now Chapter 3]). We took evidence from leading researchers and clinicians and discovered that some of the most eminent consultants worked on hunch or downright prejudice and that a woman's chance of survival, and of being surgically disfigured, greatly depended on who treated her and what those prejudices were. One surgeon favoured heroic mutilation, another preferred simple lump removal, a third opted for aggressive radiotherapy, and so on. It was as though the age of scientific appraisal had passed them by.

Indeed, it often had, and for many doctors it still does. Although things have improved, many gifted, sincere and skilful medical practitioners are surprisingly ignorant about what constitutes good scientific evidence. They do what they do because that is what they were taught in medical school, or because it is what other doctors do, or because in their experience it works. But personal experience, though beguiling, is often terribly misleading – as this book shows, with brutal clarity.

Some doctors say it is naïve to apply scientific rigour to the treatment of individual patients. Medicine, they assert, is both a science and an art. But, noble as that sounds, it is a contradiction in terms. Of course medical knowledge is finite and with any individual the complexities are almost infinite, so there is always an element of uncertainty. In practice, good medicine routinely requires good guesswork. But too often in the past many medical professionals have blurred the distinction between guessing and good evidence. Sometimes they even proclaim certainty when there is really considerable doubt. They eschew reliable data because they are not sure how to assess them.

This book explains the difference between personal experience and more complex, but better ways of distinguishing what works from what does not and what is safe from what is not. Insofar as it can, it avoids technical terms, and promotes plain English expressions like 'fair tests'. It warns that science, like everything else in human affairs, is prone to error and bias (through mistakes, vanity or – especially pernicious in medicine – the demands of commerce); but it reminds us that, even so, it is the meticulous approach of science that has created almost all of the most conspicuous advances in human knowledge. Doctors (and media-types, like me) should stop disparaging clinical research as 'trials on human guinea-pigs'; on the contrary there is a moral imperative for all practitioners to promote fair tests to their patients and for patients to participate.

This is an important book for anyone concerned about their own or their family's health, or the politics of health. Patients are often seen as the recipients of healthcare, rather than participants. The task ahead is as much for us, the lay public in whose name medicine is practised and from whose purse medical practitioners are paid, as for doctors and medical researchers. If we are passive consumers of medicine we will never drive up standards. If we prefer simplistic answers we will get pseudoscience. If we do not promote the rigorous testing of treatments we will get pointless and sometimes dangerous treatment along with the stuff that really works.

This book contains a manifesto for improving things, and patients are at its heart. But it is an important book for doctors, medical students, and researchers too – all would benefit from its lessons. In an ideal world, it would be compulsory reading for every journalist, and available to every patient, because if doctors are inadequate at weighing up scientific evidence, in general we, whose very mortality depends on this, are worse.

One thing I promise: if this subject of testing treatments is new to you, once you have read this book you will never feel quite the same about your doctor's advice again.

Nick Ross
TV and radio presenter and journalist
16 November 2005

Preface

The first edition of *Testing Treatments*, published in 2006, was inspired by a question: 'How do you ensure that research into medical treatments best meets the needs of patients?' Our collective experience – collective at that point meaning Imogen Evans, a medical doctor and former researcher and journalist, Hazel Thornton, a patient and independent lay advocate for quality in research and healthcare, and Iain Chalmers, a health services researcher – was that research often failed to address this key issue. Moreover, we were keenly aware that many medical treatments, both new and old, were not based on sound evidence. So we set out to write a book to promote more critical public assessment of the effects of treatments by encouraging patient-professional dialogue.

We were heartened by the level of interest shown in *Testing Treatments* – both in the original British Library imprint and when we made the text freely available online at www.jameslindlibrary. org – and that it appealed to both lay and professional readers. The first edition of *Testing Treatments* has been used as a teaching aid in many countries, and several full translations are available for free download from www.testingtreatments.org.

From the outset we thought of *Testing Treatments* as work in progress; there will almost always be uncertainties about the effects of treatments, whether new or old, and therefore a continuing need for all treatments to be tested properly. To do this it is essential to visit and re-visit the evidence; to review existing evidence critically and systematically before embarking on new research, and similarly to interpret new results in the light of up-to-date systematic reviews.

Embarking on the second edition of *Testing Treatments*, we three became four, with the addition of Paul Glasziou, a general practitioner and researcher with a commitment to taking account of high-quality research evidence in everyday clinical practice. We have a new publisher – Pinter & Martin, who reprinted the first edition in 2010 – and the new text is available free on line, as before, from www.testingtreatments.org. While our basic premise remains the same, the original text has been extensively revised and updated. For example, we have expanded coverage of the benefits and harms of screening in a separate chapter (Chapter 4) entitled *Earlier is not necessarily better*. And in *Regulating tests of treatments: help or hindrance?* (Chapter 9) we describe how research can become over-policed to the detriment of patients. In the penultimate chapter (Chapter 12) we ask: '*So what makes for better healthcare?*' and show how the lines of evidence can be drawn together in ways that can make a real difference to all of us. We close with our blueprint for a better future and an action plan (Chapter 13).

We hope our book will point the way to wider understanding of how treatments can and should be tested fairly and how everyone can play a part in making this happen. This is not a 'best treatments guide' to the effects of individual therapies. Rather, we highlight issues that are fundamental to ensuring that research is soundly based, properly done, able to distinguish harmful from helpful treatments, and designed to answer questions that matter to patients, the public, and health professionals.

Imogen Evans, Hazel Thornton,
Iain Chalmers, Paul Glasziou
August 2011

Introduction

'There is no way to know when our observations about complex events in nature are complete. Our knowledge is finite, Karl Popper emphasised, but our ignorance is infinite. In medicine, we can never be certain about the consequences of our interventions, we can only narrow the area of uncertainty. This admission is not as pessimistic as it sounds: claims that resist repeated energetic challenges often turn out to be quite reliable. Such "working truths" are the building blocks for the reasonably solid structures that support our everyday actions at the bedside.'

William A. Silverman. *Where's the evidence?*
Oxford: Oxford University Press, 1998, p165

Modern medicine has been hugely successful. It is hard to imagine what life must have been like without antibiotics. The development of other effective drugs has revolutionized the treatment of heart attacks and high blood pressure and has transformed the lives of many people with schizophrenia. Childhood immunization has made polio and diphtheria distant memories in most countries, and artificial joints have helped countless people to be less troubled by pain and disability. Modern imaging techniques such as ultrasound, computed tomography (CT), and magnetic resonance imaging (MRI) have helped to ensure that patients are accurately diagnosed and receive the right treatment. The diagnosis of many types of cancer used to spell a death sentence, whereas today patients regularly live with their cancers instead of dying from them. And HIV/AIDS has largely changed from a swift killer into a chronic (long-lasting) disease.

Of course many improvements in health have come about because of social and public health advances, such as piped clean water, sanitation, and better housing. But even sceptics would have difficulty dismissing the impressive impact of modern medical care. Over the past half century or so, better healthcare has made a major contribution to increased lifespan, and has improved the quality of life, especially for those with chronic conditions.[1, 2]

But the triumphs of modern medicine can easily lead us to overlook many of its ongoing problems. Even today, too much medical decision-making is based on poor evidence. There are still too many medical treatments that harm patients, some that are of little or no proven benefit, and others that are worthwhile but are not used enough. How can this be, when every year, studies into the effects of treatments generate a mountain of results? Sadly, the evidence is often unreliable and, moreover, much of the research that is done does not address the questions that patients need answered.

Part of the problem is that treatment effects are very seldom overwhelmingly obvious or dramatic. Instead, there will usually be uncertainties about how well new treatments work, or indeed whether they do more good than harm. So carefully designed fair tests – tests that set out to reduce biases and take into account the play of chance (see Chapter 6) – are necessary to identify treatment effects reliably.

The impossibility of predicting exactly what will happen when a person gets a disease or receives a treatment is sometimes called Franklin's law, after the 18th-century US statesman Benjamin Franklin, who famously noted that 'in this world nothing can be said to be certain, except death and taxes.'[3] Yet Franklin's law is hardly second nature in society. The inevitability of uncertainty is not emphasized enough in schools, nor are other fundamental concepts such as how to obtain and interpret evidence, or how to understand information about probabilities and risks. As one commentator put it: 'At school you were taught about chemicals in test tubes, equations to describe motion, and maybe something

DON'T BE TOO CERTAIN

'Through seeking we may learn and know things better. But as for certain truth, no man hath known it, for all is but a woven web of guesses.'
Xenophanes, 6th century BCE

'I am always certain about things that are a matter of opinion.'
Charlie ('Peanuts') Brown, 20th century CE

'Our many errors show that the practice of causal inference . . . remains an art. Although to assist us, we have acquired analytic techniques, statistical methods and conventions, and logical criteria, ultimately the conclusions we reach are a matter of judgement.'
Susser M. *Causal thinking in the health sciences.*
Oxford: Oxford University Press, 1983.

on photosynthesis. But in all likelihood you were taught nothing about death, risk, statistics, and the science that will kill or cure you.[4] And whereas the practice of medicine based on sound scientific evidence has saved countless lives, you would be hard pressed to find a single exhibit explaining the key principles of scientific investigation in any science museum.

And concepts of uncertainty and risk really do matter. Take, for example, the logical impossibility of 'proving a negative' – that is, showing that something does not exist, or that a treatment has no effect. This is not just a philosophical argument; it has important practical consequences too, as illustrated by experience with a combination pill called Bendectin (active ingredients doxylamine, and pyridoxine or vitamin B6). Bendectin (also marketed as Debendox and Diclectin) used to be widely prescribed to women to relieve nausea in early pregnancy. Then came claims that Bendectin caused birth defects, which were soon taken up in an avalanche of law suits. Under pressure from all the court cases, the manufacturers of Bendectin withdrew the drug from sale in 1983. Several subsequent reviews of all the evidence provided no support for a link with birth defects – it was not possible to show conclusively that there was no harm, but there was no evidence that it did cause harm. Ironically, as a result of Bendectin being withdrawn, the only drugs available to treat morning sickness in pregnant women are those for which considerably less is known about their potential to cause birth defects.[5]

The most that research can usually do is to chip away at the uncertainties. Treatments can be harmful as well as helpful. Good, well-conducted research can indicate the *probability* (or likelihood) that a treatment for a health problem will lead to benefit or harm by comparing it with another treatment or no treatment at all. Since there are always uncertainties it helps if we try to avoid the temptation to see things in black and white. And thinking in terms of probabilities is empowering.[6] People need to know the likelihood of a particular outcome of a condition – say stroke in someone with high blood pressure – the factors that affect the chance of a stroke happening, and the probability of a treatment changing the chances of a stroke happening. With enough reliable information, patients and health professionals can then work together to assess the balance between the benefits and harms of treatments. They can then choose the option that is likely to be most appropriate according to individual circumstances and patient preferences.[7]

Our aim in *Testing Treatments* is to improve communication and boost confidence, not to undermine patients' trust in health professionals. But this can only happen when patients can help themselves and their health professionals critically assess treatment options.

In Chapter 1 we briefly describe why fair tests of treatments are necessary and how some new treatments have had harmful effects that were unexpected. In Chapter 2 we describe how the hoped-for effects of other treatments have failed to materialize, and highlight the fact that many commonly used treatments have not been adequately evaluated. Chapter 3 illustrates why more intensive treatment is not necessarily better. Chapter 4 explains why screening healthy people for early indications of disease may be harmful as well as helpful. In Chapter 5 we highlight some of the many uncertainties that pervade almost every aspect of healthcare and explain how to tackle them.

Chapters 6, 7, and 8 give some 'technical details' in a non-technical way. In Chapter 6 we outline the basis for fair testing of treatments, emphasizing the importance of ensuring that like is compared with like. Chapter 7 highlights why taking into account the play of chance is essential. Chapter 8 explains why it is so important to assess all the relevant reliable evidence systematically.

Chapter 9 outlines why systems for regulating research into the effects of treatments, through research ethics committees and other bodies, can put obstacles in the way of getting good research done, and explains why regulation may therefore fail to promote the interests of patients. Chapter 10 contrasts the key differences between good, bad, and unnecessary research into the effects of treatments; it points out how research is often distorted by commercial and academic priorities and fails to address issues that are likely to make a real difference to the well-being of patients.

Chapter 11 maps what patients and the public can do to ensure better testing of treatments. In Chapter 12 we look at ways in which robust evidence from research into treatments can really make for better healthcare for individual patients. And in Chapter 13 we present our blueprint for a better future, ending with an action plan.

Each chapter is referenced with a selection of key source material, and a separate Additional Resources section is included at the end of the book (see p184). For those who wish to explore issues in more detail, a good starting point is the James Lind Library at www.jameslindlibrary.org. You will find the free electronic version of the second edition of *Testing Treatments* at a new website – Testing Treatments Interactive (www.testingtreatments.org) – where translations and other material will be added over the coming years.

We authors are committed to the principle of equitable access to effective healthcare that is responsive to people's needs. This social responsibility in turn depends on reliable and accessible information about the effects of tests and treatments derived from sound research. Because healthcare resources everywhere are limited, treatments must be based on robust evidence and used efficiently and fairly if the whole population is to stand a chance of benefiting from medical advances. It is irresponsible to waste precious resources on treatments that are of little benefit, or to throw away, without good reason, opportunities for evaluating treatments about which too little is known. Fair testing of treatments is therefore fundamentally important to enable equitable treatment choices for all of us.

We hope that you, the reader, will emerge from *Testing Treatments* sharing some of our passion for the subject and go on to ask awkward questions about treatments, identify gaps in medical knowledge, and get involved in research to find answers for the benefit of yourself and everybody else.

1 New – but is it better?

WHY FAIR TESTS OF TREATMENTS ARE NECESSARY

Without fair – unbiased – evaluations, useless or even harmful treatments may be prescribed because they are thought to be helpful or, conversely, helpful treatments may be dismissed as useless. And fair tests should be applied to all treatments, no matter what their origin or whether they are viewed as conventional or complementary/alternative. Untested theories about treatment effects, however convincing they may sound, are just not enough. Some theories have predicted that treatments would work, but fair tests have revealed otherwise; other theories have confidently predicted that treatments would not work when, in fact, tests showed that they did.

Although there is a natural tendency to think 'new' means 'improved' – just like those advertisements for washing machine detergents – when new treatments are assessed in fair tests, they are just as likely to be found worse as they are to be found better than existing treatments. There is an equally natural tendency to think that because something has been around for a long time, it must be safe and it must be effective. But healthcare is littered with the use of treatments that are based on habit or firmly held beliefs rather than evidence: treatments that often do not do any good and sometimes do substantial harm.

There is nothing new about the need for fair tests: in the 18th century James Lind used a fair test to compare six of the remedies

---

ANECDOTES ARE ANECDOTES

'Our brains seem to be hard-wired for anecdotes, and we learn most easily through compelling stories; but I am aghast that so many people, including quite a number of my friends, cannot see the pitfalls in this approach. Science knows that anecdotes and personal experiences can be fatally misleading. It requires results that are testable and repeatable. Medicine, on the other hand, can only take science so far. There is too much human variability to be sure about anything very much when it comes to individual patients, so yes there is often a great deal of room for hunch. But let us be clear about the boundaries, for if we stray over them the essence of science is quickly betrayed: corners get cut and facts and opinions intermingle until we find it hard to distinguish one from the other.'

Ross N. Foreword. In: Ernst E, ed. *Healing, hype, or harm? A critical analysis of complementary or alternative medicine.* Exeter: Societas, 2008:vi-vii.

---

then being used to treat scurvy, a disease that was killing vast numbers of sailors during long voyages. He showed that oranges and lemons, which we now know contain vitamin C, were a very effective cure.

In 1747, while serving as a ship's surgeon aboard HMS *Salisbury,* James Lind assembled 12 of his patients at similar stages of the illness, accommodated them in the same part of the ship, and ensured that they had the same basic diet. This was crucial – it created a 'level playing field' (see Chapter 6 and box in Chapter 3, p26). Lind then allocated two sailors to receive one of the six treatments that were then in use for scurvy – cider, sulphuric acid, vinegar, seawater, nutmeg, or two oranges and a lemon. The fruit won hands down. The Admiralty later ordered that lemon juice be supplied to all ships, with the result that the deadly disease had disappeared from the Royal Navy by the end of the 18th century.

Of the treatments Lind compared, the Royal College of Physicians favoured sulphuric acid while the Admiralty favoured

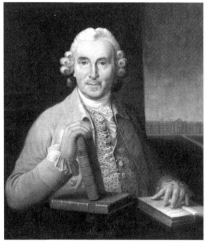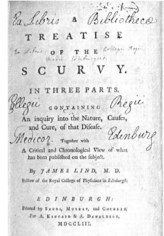

James Lind (1716-1794), Scottish naval surgeon, pictured with the books he wrote, and the title page of the most famous of these, in which he recorded a controlled trial done in 1747 showing that oranges and lemons were a more effective treatment for scurvy than five other treatments then in use (see www.jameslindlibrary.org).

vinegar – Lind's fair test showed that both authorities were wrong. Surprisingly, influential authorities are quite frequently wrong. Relying too much on opinion, habit, or precedent rather than on the results of fair tests continues to cause serious problems in healthcare (see below, and Chapter 2).

Today, uncertainties about the effects of treatments are often highlighted when doctors and other clinicians differ about the best approach for a particular condition (see Chapter 5). In addressing these uncertainties, patients and the public, as well as doctors, have an important part to play. It is in the overwhelming interest of patients, as well as professionals, that research on treatments should be rigorous. Just as health professionals must be assured that their treatment recommendations are based on sound evidence, so patients need to demand that this happens. Only by creating this critical partnership can the public have confidence in all that modern medicine has to offer (see Chapters 11, 12, and 13).

UNEXPECTED BAD EFFECTS

Thalidomide

Thalidomide is an especially chilling example of a new medical treatment that did more harm than good.[1] This sleeping pill was introduced in the late 1950s as an apparently safer alternative to the barbiturates that were regularly prescribed at that time; unlike barbiturates, overdoses of thalidomide did not lead to coma. Thalidomide was especially recommended for pregnant women, in whom it was also used to relieve morning sickness.

Then, at the beginning of the 1960s, obstetricians began to see a sharp increase in cases of severely malformed arms and legs in newborn babies. This previously rare condition results in such extremely shortened limbs that the hands and feet seem to arise directly from the body. Doctors in Germany and Australia linked these infant malformations with the fact that the mothers had taken thalidomide in early pregnancy.[2]

A TRAGIC EPIDEMIC OF BLINDNESS IN BABIES

'In the period immediately after World War II, many new treatments were introduced to improve the outlook for prematurely-born babies. Over the next few years it became painfully clear that a number of changes in caretaking practices had produced completely unexpected harmful effects. The most notable of these tragic clinical experiences was an "epidemic" of blindness, retrolental fibroplasia, in the years 1942-54. The disorder was found to be associated with the way in which supplemental oxygen had come to be used in the management of incompletely developed newborn babies. The twelve-year struggle to halt the outbreak provided a sobering demonstration of the need for planned evaluation of all medical innovations before they are accepted for general use.'

Silverman WA. Human experimentation: a guided step into the unknown. Oxford: Oxford University Press, 1985:vii-viii.

At the end of 1961, the manufacturer withdrew thalidomide. Many years later, after public campaigns and legal action, the victims began to receive compensation. The toll of these devastating abnormalities was immense – across the 46 or so countries where thalidomide was prescribed (in some countries even sold over the counter), thousands of babies were affected. The thalidomide tragedy stunned doctors, the pharmaceutical industry, and patients, and led to a worldwide overhaul of the process of drug development and licensing.[3]

Vioxx
Although drug-testing regulations have been tightened up considerably, even with the very best drug-testing practices there can be no absolute guarantee of safety. Non-steroidal anti-inflammatory drugs (NSAIDs) provide a good illustration of why vigilance in relation to drugs is needed. NSAIDs are commonly used to relieve pain and reduce inflammation in various conditions (for example, arthritis), and also to lower temperature in patients with a fever. The 'traditional' NSAIDs include many drugs that are available over the counter such as aspirin and ibuprofen. Among their side-effects, they are well known for causing irritation of the stomach and gut, leading to dyspepsia ('indigestion') and sometimes bleeding and even gastric (stomach) ulcers. Consequently, there was good reason for drug companies to see if they could develop NSAIDs that did not cause these complications.

Rofecoxib (best known by the marketing name of Vioxx, but also marketed as Ceoxx, and Ceeoxx) was introduced in 1999 as a supposedly safer alternative to the older compounds. It was soon widely prescribed. Little more than five years later Vioxx was withdrawn from the market by the manufacturer because of an increased risk of cardiovascular complications such as heart attack and stroke. So what happened?

Vioxx was approved by the US Food and Drug Administration (FDA) in 1999 for the 'relief of the signs and symptoms of osteoarthritis, for the management of acute pain in adults, and for the treatment of menstrual symptoms [that is, period pains]'. It was later approved for relief of the signs and symptoms of rheumatoid arthritis in adults and children. During development of Vioxx, drug company scientists became aware of potentially harmful effects on the body's blood clotting mechanisms which could lead to an increased risk of blood clots. Yet the generally small studies submitted to the FDA for approval purposes concentrated on evidence of Vioxx's anti-inflammatory effect and were not designed to look into the possible complications.[4]

Before the FDA approval, the company had already begun a large study mainly designed to compare gut side-effects by comparison with those of another NSAID, naproxen, in patients with rheumatoid arthritis. Once again, the study was not specifically designed to detect cardiovascular complications. Moreover, questions were later raised about conflicts of interest among members of the study's data and safety monitoring board (these boards are charged with monitoring the accumulating results of studies to see whether there is any reason for stopping the research).

Nevertheless, the results – which showed that Vioxx caused fewer episodes of stomach ulcers and gastrointestinal bleeding than naproxen – did reveal a greater number of heart attacks in the Vioxx group. Even so, the study report, published in a major medical journal, was heavily criticized. Among its flaws, the results were analyzed and presented in such a way as to downplay the seriousness of the cardiovascular risks. The journal's editor later complained that the researchers had withheld critical data on these side-effects. However, the results, submitted to the FDA in 2000, and discussed by its Arthritis Advisory Committee in 2001, eventually led the FDA to amend the safety information on Vioxx labelling in 2002 to indicate an increased risk of heart attacks and stroke.

The drug company continued to investigate other uses of Vioxx, and in 2000 embarked on a study to see whether the drug prevented colorectal (lower gut) polyps (small benign tumours that may progress to colorectal cancer). This study, which was stopped early when interim results showed that the drug was associated with an increased risk of cardiovascular complications, led to the manufacturer withdrawing Vioxx from the market in 2004. In the published report, the study's authors, who were either employed by the manufacturer or in receipt of consulting fees from the company, claimed that the cardiovascular complications only appeared after 18 months of Vioxx use. This claim was based on a flawed analysis and later formally corrected by the journal that published the report.[4] In the face of numerous subsequent legal challenges from patients, the manufacturer continues to claim that it acted responsibly at all times, from pre-approval studies to safety monitoring after Vioxx was marketed. It has also reaffirmed its belief that the evidence will show that pre-existing cardiovascular risk factors, and not Vioxx, were responsible.[5]

The Vioxx scandal shows that, half a century after thalidomide, there is still much to do to ensure that treatments are tested fairly, that the process is transparent, and that the evidence is robust. As one group of commentators put it 'Our system depends on putting patients' interests first. Collaborations between academics, practising doctors, industry, and journals are essential in advancing knowledge and improving the care of patients. Trust is a necessary element of this partnership, but the recent events have made it necessary to institute proper systems that protect the interests of patients. A renewed commitment by all those involved and the institution of these systems are the only way to extract something positive from this unfortunate affair'.[4]

Avandia

2010 saw another drug – rosiglitazone, better known by the trade name Avandia – hitting the headlines because of unwanted side-effects involving the cardiovascular system. Ten years earlier Avandia had been licensed by drug regulators in Europe and the USA as a new approach to the treatment of type 2 diabetes. This form of diabetes occurs when the body does not produce enough insulin, or when the body's cells do not react to insulin. It is far more common than type 1 diabetes, in which the body does not produce insulin at all. Type 2 diabetes, which is often associated with obesity, can usually be treated satisfactorily by modifying the diet, exercising, and taking drugs by mouth rather than by injecting insulin. The long-term complications of type 2 diabetes include an increased risk of heart attacks and strokes; the main aim of treatments is to reduce the risk of these complications.

Avandia was promoted as acting in a novel way to help the body's own insulin work more effectively and was said to be better than older drugs in controlling blood sugar levels. The focus was on the blood sugar and not on the serious complications that cause suffering and ultimately kill patients.

When Avandia was licensed, there was limited evidence of its effectiveness and no evidence about its effect on the risk of heart attacks and strokes. The drug regulators asked the manufacturer to do additional studies, but meanwhile Avandia became widely and enthusiastically prescribed worldwide. Reports of adverse cardiovascular effects began to appear and steadily mounted; by 2004 the World Health Organization was sufficiently concerned to ask the manufacturer to look again at the evidence of these complications. It did, and confirmed an increased risk.[6]

It took a further six years before the drug regulators took a really hard look at the evidence and acted. In September 2010 the US Food and Drug Administration announced that it would severely restrict the use of Avandia to patients who were unable to control their type 2 diabetes with other drugs; the same month the European Medicines Agency recommended that Avandia be withdrawn from use over the subsequent two months. Both drug regulators gave the increased risk of heart attacks and strokes as the reason for their decision. Meanwhile independently minded investigators uncovered a litany of missed opportunities for action – and, as one group of health professionals put it, a fundamental need for drug regulators and doctors to 'demand better proof before we embarked on mass medication of a large group of patients who looked to us for advice and treatment'.[7]

Mechanical heart valves

Drugs are not the only treatments that can have unexpected bad effects: non-drug treatments can pose serious risks too. Mechanical heart valves are now a standard treatment for patients with serious heart valve disease and there have been many improvements in design over the years. However, experience with a particular type of mechanical heart valve showed how one attempt to improve a design had disastrous consequences. Beginning in the early 1970s, a device known as the Björk-Shiley heart valve was introduced, but the early models were prone to thrombosis (clot formation) that impaired their function. To overcome this drawback, the design was modified in the late 1970s to reduce the possibility of clots.

The new device involved a disc held in place by two metal struts (supports), and many thousands of this new type of valve were implanted worldwide. Unfortunately, the structure of the valves was seriously flawed: one of the struts had a tendency to snap – a defect known as strut fracture – and this led to catastrophic and often fatal valve malfunction.

As it happened, strut fracture had been identified as a problem during pre-marketing tests of the device, but this was attributed to defective welding and the cause was not fully investigated. The US Food and Drug Administration (FDA) nevertheless accepted this explanation, along with the manufacturer's assurance that the lowered risk of valve thrombosis more than compensated for any risk of strut fracture. When the evidence of disastrous valve failure became only too apparent, the FDA eventually acted and forced the valve off the market in 1986, but not before hundreds of patients had died unnecessarily. Although product regulation systems have now improved to include better post-marketing patient monitoring and comprehensive patient registries, there is still a pressing need for greater transparency when new devices are introduced.[8]

TOO GOOD TO BE TRUE

Herceptin
Commercial companies are not alone in trumpeting the advantages of new treatments while down-playing drawbacks. Professional hype and enthusiastic media coverage can likewise promote benefits while ignoring potential downsides. And these downsides may include not only harmful side-effects but also diagnostic difficulties, as shown by events surrounding the breast cancer drug trastuzumab, better known by the trade name Herceptin (see also Chapter 3).

In early 2006, vociferous demands from coalitions of patients and professionals, fuelled by the pharmaceutical industry and the mass media, led the UK National Health Service to provide Herceptin for patients with early breast cancer. 'Patient pester power' triumphed – Herceptin was presented as a wonder drug (see Chapter 11).

But at that time Herceptin had only been licensed for the treatment of metastatic (widespread) breast cancer and had not been sufficiently tested for early breast cancer. Indeed, the manufacturers had only just applied for a licence for it to be used to treat early stages of the disease in a very small subset of women – those who tested positive for a protein known as HER2. And only one in five women has this genetic profile. The difficulties and costs of accurately assessing whether a patient is HER2 positive, and the potential for being incorrectly diagnosed – and therefore treated – as a 'false positive', were seldom reported by an enthusiastic but uncritical press. Nor was it emphasized that at least four out of five patients with breast cancer are not HER2 positive.[9, 10, 11, 12]

It was not until later that year that the UK's National Institute for Health and Clinical Excellence (NICE) – the organization charged with looking at evidence impartially and issuing advice – was able to recommend Herceptin as a treatment option for women with HER2 positive early breast cancer. Even then, there was an important warning. Because of mounting evidence that Herceptin could have adverse effects on heart function, NICE recommended that doctors should assess heart function before prescribing the drug, and not offer it to women with various heart problems, ranging from angina to abnormal heart rhythms. NICE judged that caution was necessary because of short-term data about side-effects, some of them serious. Long-term outcomes, both beneficial and harmful, take time to emerge.[13]

Similar pressures for use of Herceptin were being applied in other countries too. In New Zealand, for example, patient advocacy groups, the press and the media, drug companies, and politicians all demanded that breast cancer patients should be prescribed Herceptin. New Zealand's Pharmaceutical Management Agency (PHARMAC), which functions much as NICE does in the UK, similarly reviewed the evidence for use

ON BEING SUCKED INTO A MAELSTROM

In 2006, a patient in the UK, who happened to be medically trained, found herself swept along by the Herceptin tide. She had been diagnosed with HER2 positive breast cancer the preceding year.

'Prior to my diagnosis, I had little knowledge of modern management of breast cancer and, like many patients, used online resources. The Breast Cancer Care website was running a campaign to make Herceptin available to all HER2 positive women and I signed up as I simply could not understand, from the data presented on the website and in the media, why such an effective agent should be denied to women who, if they relapsed, would receive it anyway. . . . I began to feel that if I did not receive this drug then I would have very little chance of surviving my cancer! I was also contacted by the Sun newspaper who were championing the Herceptin campaign and were interested in my story, as a doctor and a "cancer victim".

At the completion of chemotherapy, I discussed Herceptin treatment with my Oncologist. He expressed concerns regarding the long-tem cardiac [heart] effects which had emerged in studies but had received very little attention on the website and from the media, especially when one considered that the drug was being given to otherwise healthy women. Also, more careful analysis of the "50% benefit" which had been widely quoted and fixed in my mind actually translated into a 4-5% benefit to me, which equally balanced the cardiac risk! So I elected not to receive the drug and will be happy with the decision even if my tumour recurs.

This story illustrates how (even) a medically trained and usually rational woman becomes vulnerable when diagnosed with a potentially life threatening illness. . . . much of the information surrounding the use of Herceptin in early breast cancer was hype generated artificially by the media and industry, fuelled by individual cases such as mine.'

Cooper J. Herceptin (rapid response). *BMJ*. Posted 29 November 2006 at www.bmj.com.

of Herceptin in early breast cancer. In June 2007, based on its review, PHARMAC decided that it was appropriate for early breast cancer patients to receive nine weeks of Herceptin, to be given at the same time as other anti-cancer drugs, rather than one after another. This nine-week course was one of three regimens then being tried around the world. PHARMAC also decided to contribute funds to an international study designed to determine the ideal length of Herceptin treatment. However, in November 2008, the newly elected government ignored PHARMAC's evidence-based decision and announced funding for a 12-month course of the drug.[14]

Numerous uncertainties remain about Herceptin – for example, about when to prescribe the drug; how long to prescribe it for; whether long-term harms might outweigh the benefits for some women; and whether the drug delays or prevents the cancer returning. A further concern that has emerged is that Herceptin, when given in combination with other breast cancer drugs such as anthracylines and cyclophosphamide, may increase the risk of patients experiencing adverse heart effects from about four patients in a hundred to about 27 patients in a hundred.[15]

KEY POINTS

- Testing new treatments is necessary because new treatments are as likely to be worse as they are to be better than existing treatments

- Biased (unfair) tests of treatments can lead to patients suffering and dying

- The fact that a treatment has been licensed doesn't ensure that it is safe

- Side-effects of treatments often take time to appear

- Beneficial effects of treatments are often overplayed, and harmful effects downplayed

2 Hoped-for effects that don't materialize

Some treatments are in use for a long time before it is realized that they can do more harm than good. Hoped-for effects may fail to materialize. In this chapter we explain how this may come about.

ADVICE ON BABIES' SLEEPING POSITION

Do not imagine that only drugs can harm – advice can be lethal too. Many people have heard of the American childcare specialist Dr Benjamin Spock, whose best-selling book *Baby and Child Care* became a bible for both professionals and parents, especially in the USA and the UK, over several decades. Yet in giving one of his pieces of well-meaning advice Dr Spock got things badly wrong. With seemingly irrefutable logic – and certainly a degree of authority – from the 1956 edition of his book until the late 1970s he argued: 'There are two disadvantages to a baby's sleeping on his back. If he vomits he's more likely to choke on the vomitus. Also he tends to keep his head turned towards the same side . . . this may flatten the side of the head . . . I think it is preferable to accustom a baby to sleeping on his stomach from the start.'

Placing babies to sleep on their front (prone) became standard practice in hospitals and was dutifully followed at home by millions of parents. But we now know that this practice – which was never rigorously evaluated – led to tens of thousands of

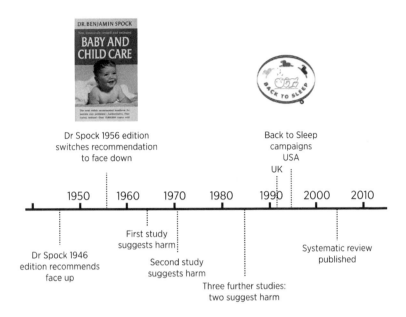

How advice on babies' sleeping position changed with time.

avoidable cot deaths.[1] Although not all cot deaths can be blamed on this unfortunate advice, there was a dramatic decline in these deaths when the practice was abandoned and advice to put babies to sleep on their backs was promoted. When clear evidence of the harmful effects of the prone sleeping position emerged in the 1980s, doctors and the media started to warn of the dangers, and the numbers of cot deaths began to fall dramatically. The message was later reinforced by concerted 'back to sleep' campaigns to remove once and for all the negative influence of Dr Spock's regrettable advice.

DRUGS TO CORRECT HEART RHYTHM ABNORMALITIES IN PATIENTS HAVING A HEART ATTACK

Dr Spock's advice may have seemed logical, but it was based on untested theory. Other examples of the dangers of doing this are not hard to find. After having a heart attack, some people develop heart rhythm abnormalities – arrhythmias. Those who do are at higher risk of death than those who don't. Since there are drugs that suppress these arrhythmias, it seemed logical to suppose that these drugs would also reduce the risk of dying after a heart attack. In fact, the drugs had exactly the opposite effect. The drugs had been tested in clinical trials, but only to see whether they reduced heart rhythm abnormalities. When the accumulated evidence from trials was first reviewed systematically in 1983, there was no evidence that these drugs reduced death rates.[2]

However, the drugs continued to be used – and continued to kill people – for nearly a decade. At the peak of their use in the late 1980s, one estimate is that they caused tens of thousands of premature deaths every year in the USA alone. They were killing more Americans every year than had been killed in action during the whole of the Vietnam war.[3] It later emerged that, for commercial reasons, the results of some trials suggesting that the drugs were lethal had never been reported (See Chapter 8, p97).[4]

DIETHYLSTILBOESTROL

At one time, doctors were uncertain whether pregnant women who had previously had miscarriages and stillbirths could be helped by a synthetic (non-natural) oestrogen called diethylstilboestrol (DES). Some doctors prescribed it and some did not. DES became popular in the early 1950s and was thought to improve a malfunction of the placenta that was believed to cause these problems. Those who used it were encouraged by anecdotal reports of women with previous miscarriages and stillbirths who, after DES treatment, had had a surviving child.

For example, one British obstetrician, consulted by a woman who had had two stillborn babies, prescribed the drug from early pregnancy onwards. The pregnancy ended with the birth of a liveborn baby. Reasoning that the woman's 'natural' capacity for successful childbearing may have improved over this time, the obstetrician withheld DES during the woman's fourth pregnancy; the baby died in the womb from 'placental insufficiency'. So, during the woman's fifth and sixth pregnancies, the obstetrician and the woman were in no doubt that DES should again be given, and the pregnancies both ended with liveborn babies. Both the obstetrician and the woman concluded that DES was a useful drug. Unfortunately, this conclusion based on anecdote was never shown to be correct in fair tests. Over the same period of time that the woman was receiving care, unbiased studies were actually being conducted and reported and they found no evidence that DES was beneficial.[5]

Although there was no evidence from fair tests that DES was helpful in preventing stillbirths, the DES story did not end there. Twenty years later evidence of harmful side-effects began to emerge when the mother of a young woman with a rare cancer of the vagina made a very important observation. The mother had been prescribed DES during pregnancy and she suggested that her daughter's cancer might have been caused by the drug.[6] This time the observation was correct, but most importantly it was *shown* to be correct. Since then, numerous studies have shown a range of serious side-effects of DES in both men and women who had been exposed to DES before they were born. These side-effects included not only an increased frequency of rare cancers but also other abnormalities of the reproductive system.

By the time it was officially declared that DES should not be used in pregnancy, several million people had been exposed to the drug. Knowing what we know now, if doctors had used the most reliable research evidence on DES available in the 1950s, many fewer would have prescribed it, because DES was never actually proved to be effective for the condition for which it had been prescribed in the first place. Tragically, this lack of evidence of benefit was widely overlooked.[7]

HORMONE REPLACEMENT THERAPY (HRT)

In women going through the menopause, hormone replacement therapy (HRT) is very effective in reducing the distressing hot flushes that are commonly experienced, and there is some evidence that it may help to prevent osteoporosis (bone thinning). Gradually, more and more beneficial effects were claimed for HRT, including prevention of heart attacks and stroke. And millions of

NO WONDER SHE WAS CONFUSED

In January 2004, a hysterectomy patient wrote this letter to *The Lancet:*

'In 1986 I had a hysterectomy because of fibroids. The surgeon also removed my ovaries and found that I had endometriosis as well. Because I was then only 45 years old and would have had an immediate menopause, I was put onto hormone replacement therapy (HRT). The first year I took conjugated oestrogens (Premarin), but from 1988 until 2001 I had oestrogen implants every 6 months, given to me privately by the surgeon who did the operation. I was always a little dubious about having the treatment, since I felt I just did not have control over things once the implant was done, and also after several years had many headaches. Apart from that I felt very fit.

However, my surgeon assured me that HRT had so many advantages and that it suited me, which I agreed with. As time went on, HRT was reported to have more and more benefits and was not just the cosmetic drug it seemed to have been used for in its early years. It was now good for the heart, osteoporosis, and part defence against strokes. Every time I visited my surgeon, he seemed to have more evidence about the advantages of taking HRT.

My surgeon retired in 2001 and I went to my National Health Service doctor. What a shock! He told me the exact opposite of my private surgeon – that it would be a good idea to come off HRT: it could increase the risk of heart disease, strokes, and breast cancer, and be the cause of headaches. I did have one more implant and then went onto Premarin for a short while, but since then I have not used HRT for about 8 months. My doctor said it would be my decision whether to stay on it or not. I was so confused . . .

I cannot understand how HRT and all its wonderful advantages can be reversed in such a short space of time. How can a layman like myself come to a clear decision? I have spent many hours discussing and thinking about whether I should have stayed on HRT, although so far I have not suffered many ill effects. I am very confused about the whole issue and I am sure other women feel the same.'

Huntingford CA. Confusion over benefits of hormone replacement therapy. *Lancet* 2004;363:332.

women, advised by their doctors, began using HRT for longer because of claims of these and other extra benefits. However, the basis of these claims was very shaky.

Take heart attacks alone. For over 20 years, women were told that HRT would reduce their risk of this serious condition – in fact the advice was based on the results of biased (unfair) studies (see Chapter 1 and Chapter 6). Then, in 1997, there was a warning that the advice might be wrong: researchers from Finland and the UK reviewed, systematically, the results of well-conducted studies.[8] They found that, far from reducing heart disease, HRT might actually increase it. Some prominent commentators dismissed this conclusion, but its tentative result has now been confirmed by two large well-conducted trials. Had the effects of HRT been assessed properly when it was first introduced, women would not have been misinformed and many of them would not have died prematurely. To make matters worse, we now know that HRT increases the risk of stroke and of developing breast cancer.[9]

Overall, HRT continues to be a valuable treatment for women with menopausal symptoms.[10] However, it is tragic that it was so heavily promoted specifically as a way of reducing heart attacks and stroke. Although the increased chance of these serious conditions is modest, the total number of women affected is very large indeed because HRT has been so widely prescribed.

EVENING PRIMROSE OIL FOR ECZEMA

Even if inadequately assessed treatments do not kill or harm, they can waste money. Eczema is a distressing skin complaint affecting both children and adults. The skin lesions are both unsightly and very itchy. Although the use of steroid creams helps in this condition, there were concerns about the side-effects of these treatments, such as thinning of the skin. In the early 1980s a natural plant oil extract – evening primrose oil – emerged as a possible alternative with few side-effects.[11] Evening primrose oil contains an essential fatty acid called gamma-linolenic acid (GLA) and there were plausible reasons for using it. One suggestion, for example, was that the way in which GLA was transformed within

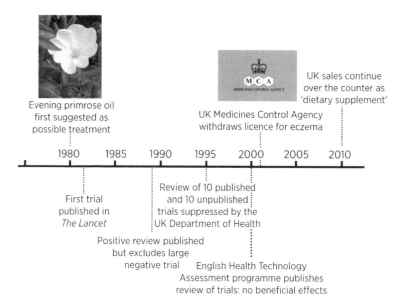

Evening primrose oil first suggested as possible treatment

UK Medicines Control Agency withdraws licence for eczema

UK sales continue over the counter as 'dietary supplement'

1980   1985   1990   1995   2000   2005   2010

First trial published in *The Lancet*

Review of 10 published and 10 unpublished trials suppressed by the UK Department of Health

Positive review published but excludes large negative trial

English Health Technology Assessment programme publishes review of trials: no beneficial effects

Timeline for evidence about and use of evening primrose oil in eczema.

the body (metabolized) was impaired in patients with eczema. So, theoretically, giving GLA supplements should help. Borage oil, also known as starflower oil, contains even higher amounts of GLA and this was also recommended for eczema.

GLA was believed to be safe but was it effective? Numerous studies were done to find out but they gave conflicting results. And the published evidence was heavily influenced by studies sponsored by the companies making the supplements. In 1995, the Department of Health in the UK requested researchers unconnected with the manufacturers of evening primrose oil to review 20 published and unpublished studies. No evidence of benefit was found. The Department never made the report public because the manufacturers of the drug objected. But five years later another systematic review of both evening primrose oil and borage oil by the same researchers – this time it was published – showed that in the largest and most complete studies there was no convincing evidence that these treatments worked.[12]

There was one unturned stone – perhaps GLA only worked in very high doses. In 2003, even this claim was knocked on the head by a carefully conducted fair test.[13] Ironically, by the time these results were published, the UK Medicines Control Agency (MCA, which subsequently became the Medicines and Healthcare products Regulatory Agency, MHRA) had finally, in October 2002, withdrawn the product licences for two major evening primrose oil preparations because there was no evidence that they worked.

Nevertheless, since no concerns were expressed about the safety of evening primrose oil, it is still widely available over the counter as a 'dietary supplement' for various conditions. Regarding its use for eczema, claims of effectiveness are couched in vague terms such as 'people with eczema may find relief', 'may be helpful' and 'has certain medicinal properties that may act as an anti-inflammatory for conditions such as eczema'.

KEY POINTS

- Neither theory nor professional opinion is a reliable guide to safe, effective treatments

- Just because a treatment is 'established' does not mean it does more good than harm

- Even if patients do not suffer from inadequately tested treatments, using them can waste individual and community resources

---

3 More is not necessarily better

A popular misconception is that if a treatment is good then more of it must be better. This is simply not true – indeed more can be worse. Finding the 'right' dose – where benefits are high and adverse effects (side-effects) are low – is a challenge common to all treatments. As the dose is increased, beneficial effects reach a plateau, but adverse effects usually increase. So 'more' may decrease the actual benefit, or even cause overall harm.

Diuretics (water tablets) are a good example: in low doses they lower blood pressure and have few adverse effects. A higher dose does not lower blood pressure any further but does lead to unwanted effects, such as excess urination, impotence and increased blood sugar. Similarly, aspirin in low doses – between a quarter and a half of a standard tablet per day – helps to prevent strokes, and with very few adverse effects. However, while several aspirin tablets per day might relieve a headache, they will not prevent any more strokes and will increase the risk of stomach ulcers.

This principle of the 'right dose' extends beyond drug therapy to many other treatments, including surgery.

INTENSIVE TREATMENTS FOR BREAST CANCER

The therapies advocated for breast cancer – so often in the news – provide some especially valuable lessons about the dangers of assuming that more intensive treatments are necessarily beneficial.

WE DO THINGS BECAUSE ...

'We [doctors] do things, because other doctors do so and we don't want to be different, so we do so; or because we were taught so [by teachers, fellows and residents (junior doctors)]; or because we were forced [by teachers, administrators, regulators, guideline developers] to do so, and think that we must do so; or because patient wants so, and we think we should do so; or because of more incentives [unnecessary tests (especially by procedure oriented physicians) and visits], we think we should do so; or because of the fear [by the legal system, audits] we feel that we should do so [so-called 'covering oneself']; or because we need some time [to let nature take its course], so we do so; finally and more commonly, that we have to do something [justification] and we fail to apply common sense, so we do so.'

Parmar MS. We do things because (rapid response). *BMJ*. Posted 1 March 2004 at www.bmj.com.

Throughout the 20th century and into the 21st, women with breast cancer have both demanded and endured some exceedingly brutal and distressing treatments. Some of these treatments – surgical and medical – far exceeded what was actually required to tackle the disease. But they were also unquestionably popular with some patients as well as their doctors. Patients were convinced that the more radical or toxic the therapy, the more likely the disease would be 'conquered'. It has taken doctors and patients who have been prepared to challenge orthodox views of the condition many years to begin to turn the tide of mistaken belief. They not only had to produce reliable evidence to banish the myth that 'more is better', but also suffer the ridicule of their peers and the resistance of eminent practitioners.

Today, fear, coupled with the belief that more must be better, still drives treatment choices, even when there is no evidence of

---

DRASTIC TREATMENT IS NOT ALWAYS THE BEST

'It is very easy for those of us treating cancer to imagine that better results are due to a more drastic treatment. Randomized trials comparing drastic treatment with less drastic treatment are vital in order to protect patients from needless risk and the early or late side effects of unnecessarily aggressive treatment. The comparison is ethical because those who are denied possible benefit are also shielded from possible unnecessary harm – and nobody knows which it will turn out to be in the end.'

Brewin T in Rees G, ed. *The friendly professional: selected writings of Thurstan Brewin.* Bognor Regis: Eurocommunica, 1996.

---

benefit over simpler approaches, and where known harms are considerable, including the possibility of death from the treatment itself. For example, this mindset still prompts some patients and their doctors to opt for 'traditional' mutilating surgery. Others choose high-dose chemotherapy, with its well known unpleasant and painful side-effects, or Herceptin, which can cause serious heart problems (see Chapter 1), even when simpler treatments would be sufficient. How can this be?

Mutilating surgery

Until the middle of the 20th century, surgery was the main treatment for breast cancer. This was based on the belief that the cancer progressed in a slow and orderly manner, first spreading from the tumour in the breast to local lymph nodes, in the armpit, for example. Consequently it was reasoned that the more radical and prompt the surgery for the tumour, the better the chance of halting the spread of the cancer. Treatment was by extensive 'local' surgery – that is, surgery on or near the breast. It may have been called local, but a radical mastectomy was anything but – it involved removing large areas of chest muscle and much lymph node tissue from the armpits as well as the breast itself.

THE CLASSICAL (HALSTED) RADICAL MASTECTOMY

The radical mastectomy, devised in the late 19th century by William Halsted, was the most commonly performed operation for breast cancer until the third quarter of the 20th century. As well as removing all of the breast, the surgeon cut away the pectoralis major muscle covering the chest wall. The smaller pectoralis minor muscle was also removed to allow the surgeon easier access to the armpit (axilla) to clear out the lymph nodes and surrounding fat.

EXTENDED RADICAL MASTECTOMIES

The belief that 'more is better' led radical surgeons to carry out even more extensive operations, in which chains of lymph nodes under the collarbone and the internal mammary nodes under the breastbone were also removed. To get at the internal mammary nodes several ribs were removed and the breastbone was split with a chisel. Not content with that, some surgeons went so far as to remove the arm on the affected side and cut out various glands throughout the body (adrenals, pituitary, ovaries) to suppress the production of hormones that were believed to 'fuel' the spread of the tumour.

If a woman survived such operations she was left with a severely mutilated ribcage, which was difficult to conceal under any clothing. If surgery had been carried out on the left side, only a thin layer of skin remained to cover the heart.

Adapted from Lerner BH, *The breast cancer wars: hope, fear and the pursuit of a cure in twentieth-century America.* New York; Oxford University Press, 2003.

Nevertheless, some thoughtful breast cancer specialists noted that these increasingly mutilating operations did not seem to be having any impact on death rates from breast cancer. So, they put forward a different theory – that breast cancer, rather than spreading from the breast through the nearby lymph nodes, was in fact a systemic (that is, widespread) disease from the outset. In other words, they reasoned that cancer cells must already be present elsewhere in the body at the time the breast lump was detected (see below). If so, they suggested, removal of the tumour with an adequate margin of normal tissue, plus a course of local radiotherapy, would be both kinder to the woman and might be as effective as radical surgery. The introduction of 'systemic therapies' at about this time – that is, treatments that would deal with production or development of cancer cells elsewhere in the body – was also based on this new theory of breast cancer spread.

As a direct result of this new way of thinking, doctors advocated more limited surgery known as lumpectomy – that is, removal of the tumour and a margin of surrounding normal tissue. Lumpectomy was followed by radiotherapy, and in some women by chemotherapy. But supporters of lumpectomy encountered huge resistance to comparing the new approach with radical surgery. Some doctors believed very firmly in one or other approach and patients clamoured for one or other treatment. The result was a prolonged delay in producing the crucial evidence about the merits and harms of the proposed new treatment compared with the old.

Nevertheless, despite these difficulties, the surgical excesses were eventually challenged, both by surgeons who were unwilling to continue in the face of questionable benefits for their patients, and by outspoken women who were unwilling to undergo mutilating operations.

In the mid-1950s, George Crile, an American surgeon, led the way by going public with his concerns about the 'more is better' approach. Believing that there was no other tactic to stir doctors into thinking critically, Crile appealed to them in an article in the popular *Life* magazine.[1] He hit the right note: the debate within the medical profession was now out in the open rather than confined to academic circles. Then another US surgeon, Bernard Fisher, working together with colleagues in other specialties, devised a series of rigorous experiments to study the biology of cancer. Their results suggested that cancer cells could indeed travel widely through the bloodstream, even before the primary cancer was discovered. So, aggressive surgery made little sense if the cancer was already present elsewhere in the body.

Whereas Crile had used his clinical judgment to advocate and employ less radical local therapies, Fisher and a growing group of researchers collaborated in a more formal and rigorous approach. They sought to prove or disprove the value of radical surgery by the best-known unbiased (fair) method – randomized trials (see Chapter 6). They reasoned that by doing such studies the medical community and the general public might be convinced one way or the other. In 1971, the outspoken Fisher also declared that surgeons had an ethical and moral responsibility to test their theories by conducting such trials. And certainly, the 20-year follow-up of Fisher's trials showed that – as measured by the risk of early death – no advantage could be demonstrated for radical mastectomy compared with lumpectomy followed by radiation therapy.[2]

RANDOM ALLOCATION – A SIMPLE EXPLANATION

'Randomisation is to minimise bias and ensure that the patients in each treatment group are as similar as possible in all known and unknown factors. This will ensure that any differences found between the groups in the outcome(s) of interest are due to differences in treatment effect and not differences between the patients receiving each of the treatments.

It removes the chance that a clinician will consciously or unconsciously allocate one treatment to a particular type of patient and the other treatment to another type, or that a certain kind of patient will choose one treatment whilst another kind will choose the other.'

Harrison J. Presentation to Consumers' Advisory Group for Clinical Trials, 1995.

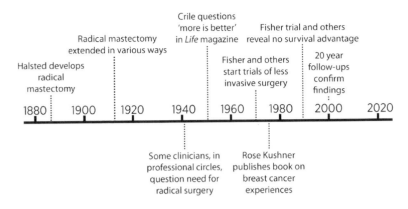

Challenging the 'more is better' approach in breast cancer surgery.

Randomized trials (see Chapter 6) were also done by researchers in other countries comparing breast-conserving therapy with radical mastectomy, for example by Hedley Atkins and colleagues in the UK in the early 1960s and later by Veronesi and colleagues in Italy. The overall picture confirmed Fisher's results: that there was no evidence that radical mastectomy led to longer survival, even after 20 years of follow-up.[3] Other randomized trials, in Sweden and Italy as well as the UK and the USA, were done to compare many other forms of treatment – for example, radiation therapy after surgery compared with surgery alone, and short-term compared with long-term chemotherapies.

Overall, results from these early trials and from detailed laboratory studies supported the theory that breast cancer was indeed a systemic disease, with cancer cells spreading via the bloodstream before a breast lump was detectable.[4] Worldwide, more and more doctors became convinced by the mounting evidence that radical surgery was doing more harm than good. And in the last decades of the 20th century attitudes of patients and the public began changing too. Spearheaded by the work of patient activists such as Rose Kushner (see Chapter 11) in the USA and elsewhere, better informed patient groups came together from around the globe to challenge the 'more is better' approach to surgery and the medical paternalism that often went with it.

This widespread activity of both patients and health

professionals effectively challenged the surgical excesses of the past almost everywhere. Incredibly, however, there are still some reports of unnecessary and mutilating breast surgery being done – for example, in 2003, over 150 radical breast operations were carried out in Japan.[5]

By 1985, the sheer volume of breast cancer trials on all aspects of treatment made it very difficult for people to keep sufficiently up to date with the results. To address this problem, Richard Peto and his colleagues in Oxford drew together all the trial findings in the first of a series of systematic reviews (see Chapter 8) of all the information about all of the women who had participated in the many studies.[6] Systematic reviews of treatments for breast cancer are now updated and published regularly.[7, 8]

Bone marrow transplantation

However, the demise of mutilating surgery did not spell the end of the 'more is better' mindset – far from it. During the last two decades of the 20th century, a new treatment approach, involving high-dose chemotherapy followed by bone marrow transplantation or 'stem cell rescue', was introduced. A report in the *New York Times* in 1999 summed up the reasoning behind this approach:

> 'Doctors remove some bone marrow or red blood cells from the patient, then load her with huge amounts of toxic drugs, quantities that destroy the bone marrow. The hope is that the high doses will eliminate the cancer and that the saved bone marrow, when returned to the body, will grow back quickly enough so that the patient does not die from infection. A version of the procedure, using donations of bone marrow, had long been established as effective for blood cancer, but solely because the cancer was in the marrow that was being replaced. The use of the treatment for breast cancer involved a completely different – and untested – reasoning.'[9]

In the USA especially, thousands of desperate women pressed for this very unpleasant treatment from doctors and hospitals, even though as many as five out of 100 patients died from the treatment. Many thousands of dollars were spent, including some from the patients' own pockets. Eventually, some patients were reimbursed by their health insurance companies, who caved in to pressure to do so, despite the lack of evidence that the treatment was useful. Many hospitals and clinics became rich on the proceeds. In 1998, one hospital corporation made $128 million, largely from its cancer centres providing bone marrow transplants. For US doctors it was a lucrative source of income and prestige and it provided a rich field for producing publications. Insistent patient demand fuelled the market. Competition from private US hospitals to provide the treatments was intense, with cut-price offers advertised. In the 1990s, even US academic medical centres trying to recruit patients for clinical trials were offering this treatment. These questionable programmes had become a 'cash cow' for the cancer services.

Unrestricted access to such unproven treatments had another serious downside: there were not enough patients available to

---

THE STRUGGLE FOR UNBIASED EVIDENCE

Researchers expected it would take about three years to enrol about 1,000 women in the two studies. Instead it took seven years . . . That is not so surprising . . . Patients in the clinical trials must sign a consent form spelling out their grim prognosis and stating that there is no evidence that bone marrow transplants are any better than standard therapies. To enter the trial, you have to face these realities, which is never easy. But if the patient has a transplant outside a trial with a control group of patients, known as a randomized trial, enthusiastic doctors may tell her that a transplant could save her life. Although patients have a right to the truth, they understandably are not going to go to doctors who take away hope.

Adapted from Kolata G, Eichenwald K. Health business thrives on
unproven treatment, leaving science behind.
New York Times Special Report, 2 October 1999.

---

take part in trials comparing these treatments with standard therapies. As a result it took far longer than anticipated to get reliable answers.

But despite the difficulties of obtaining unbiased evidence in the face of such pressures, some clinical trials were carried out and other evidence reviewed critically. And by 2004, a systematic review of the accumulated results of conventional chemotherapy compared with high-dose chemotherapy followed by bone marrow transplantation, as a general treatment for breast cancer, failed to reveal any convincing evidence that it was useful.[10, 11]

DARE TO THINK ABOUT DOING LESS

So, more is not always better – and this message remains important. Today, in women with metastatic (widespread) breast cancer, there is considerable enthusiasm for treatments such as Herceptin (see above and Chapter 1). Yet, at best, Herceptin offers these patients a small chance of a longer life – measured sometimes only in days or weeks – at the expense of serious side-effects, or sometimes even death from the treatment itself.[12,13] This tendency to over-treat is also evident at the other end of the breast cancer spectrum. For example, excessive and often unnecessary treatments have been used in women with pre-cancerous conditions such as ductal carcinoma in situ (DCIS) detected by breast screening (see Chapter 4), when DCIS might never go on to cause a woman a problem in her lifetime if left untreated. Meanwhile, the need for routine surgery to remove lymph nodes in the armpit, which risks unpleasant complications affecting the arm such as lymphoedema (see Chapter 5), is being increasingly challenged, since its addition to other treatments does not seem to improve survival.[14]

KEY POINT

- More intensive treatment is not necessarily beneficial, and can sometimes do more harm than good

---

4 Earlier is not necessarily better

In the first three chapters we have shown how treatments that are inadequately tested can cause serious harm. Here we turn our attention to screening apparently well people for early signs of illness. Screening sounds so sensible – how better to ward off serious consequences of disease and stay healthy? While screening is helpful for several conditions, screening can harm as well as help.

In this chapter we draw on various disease examples to show why earlier diagnosis can be but is not always better; why many types of screening are of no, or uncertain, benefit; and how the

---

FROM PERSON TO PATIENT

Screening will inevitably turn some people who test 'positive' into patients – a transformation not to be undertaken lightly. 'If a patient asks a medical practitioner for help, the doctor does the best possible. The doctor is not responsible for defects in medical knowledge. If, however, the practitioner initiates screening procedures the doctor is in a very different situation. The doctor should, in our view, have conclusive evidence that screening can alter the natural history of the disease in a significant proportion of those screened.'

Cochrane AL, Holland WW. Validation of screening procedures. *British Medical Bulletin* 1971;27:3-8.

---

benefits of screening have often been oversold and the harms downplayed or ignored.

Screening healthy people should never be undertaken lightly; there are always important downsides that should make us cautious. Screening is a medical intervention. Not only that, the offer of screening is in itself an intervention. Even someone who chooses to decline screening will be left with a nagging doubt about whether they have made the 'right' decision – that is human nature. *Not* being offered screening in the first place is very different.

At best, screening should only be offered to the healthy people it seeks to reassure or treat if there is sound evidence that: (a) it will do more good than harm at an affordable cost; and (b) it will be delivered as part of a good quality and well-run programme (see below).[1]

Screening is much more than a 'one-off' test. People invited for screening need sufficient unbiased, relevant information so that they can decide whether to accept the offer or not – that is, they need to know what they are letting themselves in for (see below).[2]

One way of thinking about screening is like this:

Screening = a test plus an effective management strategy

LESSONS FROM NEUROBLASTOMA SCREENING

Experience with screening for neuroblastoma – a rare cancer that mainly occurs in young children – is instructive in several ways. This tumour affects nerve cells in various parts of the body. Survival rates for affected children depend on factors such as which part of the body is affected, how widely the tumour has spread when diagnosed, and the age of the child. The overall five-year survival rate of children aged one to four years at diagnosis is around 55%.[3] A curious feature of neuroblastoma is that it is one of the few types of cancer that sometimes disappears completely without treatment – a phenomenon called spontaneous regression.[4]

Neuroblastoma was a tempting target for screening for four

reasons: (1) children who are diagnosed before the age of one year are known to have a better outlook than those who are diagnosed later; (2) children with advanced disease fare much worse than those with early disease; (3) there is a simple and cheap screening test that can be carried out by blotting wet nappies and measuring substances in the urine; and (4) the test detects nine out of ten children with neuroblastoma.[5]

Mass screening of infants for neuroblastoma at six months of age was first introduced in Japan in 1985 without the benefit of unbiased (fair) evidence from clinical trials. During the first three years of nationwide screening over 337 infants were diagnosed, 97% of whom were alive in 1990 following treatment. But 20 years later there was no evidence that neuroblastoma screening had reduced the number of children dying from this cancer. How could that be?

When the evidence on which screening had been introduced and promoted in Japan was scrutinized it turned out that there were serious flaws – but a ready explanation. The impressive 97% survival figure illustrates the effect of something known technically as 'length-time bias' – meaning that screening works best at picking up slowly developing conditions (slow-growing tumours in this case). By contrast, fast-growing tumours are less likely to be picked up by screening but will lead to clinical signs in the infant – for example, a swelling in the abdomen – which will rapidly be brought to a doctor's attention. These fast growing tumours are potentially much more serious than slow-growing ones. Slow-growing neuroblastomas usually have a good outcome, including spontaneous regression (see above).[6]

So the 337 cases diagnosed by screening would mostly have had a good outcome anyway and would not have included infants with the worst potential outcomes. And of course screening would have picked up some neuroblastomas that would have disappeared naturally. Without screening no-one would ever have known that these tumours existed; with screening, this over-diagnosis turned the affected infants into patients, who then went on to be exposed to unnecessary harms associated with treatment.

In addition, the encouraging results from small studies that had led to the nationwide screening in Japan had initially

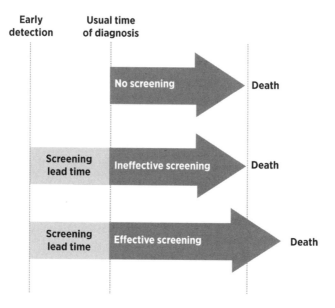

Living longer with a disease label.

been analyzed by looking at length of survival from the date of diagnosis of neuroblastoma, not at length of survival from date of birth. This is important because diagnosing a disease earlier does not automatically make patients live longer – they merely live for a longer time with the disease 'label'. Put another way, survival appears longer because the 'disease clock' starts earlier. This is an example of another sort of bias known as 'lead-time bias' – and it can be overcome by analysing the results by date of birth instead of age at diagnosis.

By contrast, when unbiased evidence was obtained from clinical trials done in Canada and Germany, involving about three million children in all, researchers were unable to detect any benefit from screening, but there were obvious harms.[7] These included unjustified surgery and chemotherapy, both of which can have serious unwanted effects. In the light of this evidence, infant screening for neuroblastoma in Japan was stopped in 2004.

Meanwhile the infants of New South Wales in Australia were largely spared from neuroblastoma screening, which had been planned in the 1980s after the encouraging early Japanese studies.

DON'T ASSUME EARLY DETECTION IS WORTHWHILE

'Screening for neuroblastoma illustrates how easily one can fall into the trap of assuming that because a disease can be detected early, screening must be worthwhile . . . The two studies demonstrate how neuroblastoma screening was not only worthless, but led to "over-diagnosis" and must have identified tumours that would have spontaneously regressed. Both studies mentioned children in the screened group suffering severe complications due to the treatment . . . Hopefully these lessons will be learned when considering the implementation of other screening programmes – for example screening for prostate cancer.'

Morris JK. Screening for neuroblastoma in children.
Journal of Medical Screening 2002;9:56.

But the Japanese results, as mentioned above, showed longer survival from date of diagnosis for the screened infants; survival from date of birth had not been analyzed. So, an Australian specialist stepped in and re-analyzed the Japanese results from dates of birth of the infants rather than from dates of diagnosis – this analysis did not show any difference in the survival rates of the screened and unscreened infants. This convinced the New South Wales authorities to abandon their screening programme, thereby saving the infants from unnecessary harms and the health service from unnecessary expense.

WEIGHING BENEFITS AND HARMS

There are many examples of beneficial screening. Perhaps the most widely used in adults is the checking of risk factors for heart disease and stroke that is routinely done in primary care. There is good evidence that high blood pressure, high blood cholesterol levels, and tobacco smoking increase the risk of these diseases, and that identifying, advising, and treating people with such risk factors can prevent heart attacks and strokes.

Phenylketonuria screening: clearly beneficial

Newborn babies are routinely screened for an inherited disease called phenylketonuria (PKU). Babies with PKU are unable to process phenylalanine, a substance which is present in everyday foods such as milk, meat, fish, and eggs. If the condition is left untreated, phenylalanine accumulates in the blood and leads to serious, irreversible, brain damage. PKU testing involves taking a few drops of blood from the baby's heel, which are analyzed in a laboratory. If this 'heel prick test' is positive, and the diagnosis is confirmed by further tests, babies are treated with a special diet to help them develop normally.

Abdominal aortic aneurysm screening: proceed with care

At the other end of the age spectrum, abdominal aortic aneurysm screening can also be beneficial. The aorta is the main blood vessel in the body, running from the heart through the chest and abdomen. In some people the wall of the aorta in the abdomen weakens as they become older and the vessel starts to expand – this is an aneurysm, a condition that seldom gives rise to symptoms and is most common in men aged 65 and over. Large aneurysms can eventually rupture and leak without warning, often causing death.[8]

This evidence concerning the frequency of aneurysms in older men can be used as the basis for introducing a screening programme. In the UK, for example, men (but not women) as they turn 65 are being offered a screening ultrasound scan. The scans can show the large aneurysms so that these men can receive specialist advice and treatment, usually surgery. Men with smaller aneurysms are monitored by further scans, and those whose aorta is not enlarged need not be screened again. The quality of the screening and the surgery is crucially important. Aneurysm surgery is a major procedure and if complication rates are high then more men would be harmed than helped.

Breast cancer screening:
well established but remains contentious

Since routine breast screening with mammography is well established in many countries one could well assume that mammographic screening must be based on sound evidence of benefits outweighing harms. As one US public health expert remarked in 2010: 'No screening test has ever been more carefully studied. In the past 50 years, more than 600,000 women have participated in 10 randomized trials, each involving approximately 10 years of follow-up'. But he went on to say 'Given this extraordinary research effort, it is ironic that screening mammography continues to be one of the most contentious issues within the medical community'.[9]

Why is mammographic screening so contentious? A fundamental reason is that it has been 'sold' to women as a sensible thing to do by those providing screening and by patient groups. The information provided to women who are invited for breast screening emphasizes the benefits while glossing over the harms, limitations, and consequences.[10] Yet mammography not only leads to early diagnosis but also, much as with prostate cancer (see below), to diagnosis of cancers that would never have become apparent in a patient's lifetime. And inevitably there will be false-positive results too.

The most reliable evidence comes from reviewing, systematically, the results of clinical trials in which women have been randomly allocated to screening or no screening. And the results make for interesting reading. They show that if 2,000 women are screened regularly for ten years, one will benefit from screening, as she will avoid dying from breast cancer. But at the same time, ten healthy women will, as a consequence of screening, become 'cancer patients' and will be treated unnecessarily. Mammography in these women has in fact detected lesions that are so slow-growing (or even not growing at all) that they would never have developed into a real cancer. These healthy women will go on to have either part of their breast removed, or even the whole breast, and will often receive radiotherapy and sometimes chemotherapy.[11]

Furthermore, 200 screened women out of 2,000 will experience a false alarm, and the psychological strain until the woman knows whether it was cancer, and even afterwards, can be severe. And mammography is often promoted to women alongside advice on breast self-examination or breast awareness, when both these methods have also been shown to result in more harm than benefit.[12]

A British public health expert noted that the potential for individual benefit from mammography is very small. He remarked: 'this is not widely understood. In part this is due to obfuscation from organisers of mammography services assuming that a positive emphasis is needed to ensure reasonable compliance [with screening]'. Assessing the available evidence in 2010, he commented: 'Mammography does save lives, more effectively among older women, but does cause some harm.' The harms he is referring to are overdiagnosis and false positives. Critically, he observed that full examination of all the individual results from recent screening studies had yet to be examined dispassionately.[13] While such an impartial evaluation is awaited, women continue to be invited for mammographic screening. At the very least, they need to be given sufficiently balanced information to enable them to decide (together with their family and their doctor if they wish), whether to attend for screening – or not.

Prostate cancer screening:
clear harms with uncertain benefits

Prostate cancer is the second most common cancer in men worldwide,[14] and broadly falls into two types. Some men have an aggressive form of the disease; these dangerous cancers spread rapidly and the death rate is high. But many men have slow-growing cancers that would never progress to cause a danger to health during a man's lifetime. Ideally, a screening test would detect the dangerous cancers – with the hope that they could be treated – but not the slow-growing ones. The reason is that treatment of any sort of prostate cancer risks distressing side-effects such as incontinence and impotence – a heavy price to pay if the cancer would not have caused problems in the first place.[15]

Blood levels of a substance called prostate-specific antigen (PSA) are raised in most men with prostate cancer. However, there is no clear cut-off level that will distinguish between men who have cancer and those who do not,[16] and as many as one in five men with clinically significant cancers will have normal PSA levels. Moreover, despite its name, PSA is anything but 'specific'

OVERDIAGNOSING PROSTATE CANCER

'Prostate cancer has been described as the *par excellence* example of overdiagnosis. This does *not* mean that there are not men whose lives are saved from early death from prostate cancer by early diagnosis. But . . . we have little way of knowing in advance *which* men will benefit from screening and which will be unnecessarily treated, often with serious adverse consequences to their life. The fundamental problem is that by screening and testing for prostate cancer we are finding many more prostate cancers than we ever did before, and strange as it may seem, many of these cancers would never become life threatening. In the past these men would never have known they had prostate cancer, they would go on to die of something else, dying *with* their prostate cancer, rather than *because of* it. By finding all these prostate cancers that are indolent we are giving many more men a prostate cancer diagnosis than ever before. Hence the term "overdiagnosis". This is the core dilemma that each man contemplating being tested faces.'

Chapman S, Barratt A, Stockler M. Let sleeping dogs lie? *What men should know before getting tested for prostate cancer.* Sydney: Sydney University Press, 2010: p25

– for example, non-cancerous prostate tumours, infections, and even some over-the-counter pain-killers can cause raised PSA levels. On these grounds alone, PSA clearly has serious limitations as a screening test.

Yet routine PSA testing of healthy men has been enthusiastically promoted for prostate cancer screening by professional and patient groups and by companies selling the tests, and has been widely adopted in many countries. The pro-PSA-screening lobby has been especially vocal in the USA, where it is estimated that, each year, 30 million men are tested, believing that this is the sensible thing to do. So what is the evidence that earlier detection of prostate cancer with PSA screening improves a man's outcome;

DISCOVERER OF PSA SPEAKS OUT

'The test's popularity has led to a hugely expensive public health disaster. It's an issue I am painfully familiar with – I discovered PSA in 1970. . . .

Americans spend an enormous amount testing for prostate cancer. The annual bill for PSA screening is at least $3 billion, with much of it paid for by Medicare and the Veterans Administration.

Prostate cancer may get a lot of press, but consider the numbers: American men have a 16 percent lifetime chance of receiving a diagnosis of prostate cancer but only a 3 percent chance of dying from it. That's because the majority of prostate cancers grow slowly. In other words, men lucky enough to reach old age are much more likely to die with prostate cancer than to die of it.

Even then the test is hardly more effective than a coin toss. As I've been trying to make clear for many years now, PSA testing can't detect prostate cancer and, more important, it can't distinguish between the two types of prostate cancer – the one that will kill you and the one that won't.'

Ablin RJ. The great prostate mistake. *New York Times*, 10 March 2010.

and what is known about harms associated with testing?

High-quality evidence about the benefits and harms of PSA screening is now becoming available. In 2010, the results from all relevant trials were systematically reviewed. This assessment showed that, although PSA screening increased the likelihood of being diagnosed with prostate cancer (as would be expected), there was no evidence of an impact on either the rate of death from the cancer or the overall death rate.[17]

So, is the tide turning against PSA screening? Richard Ablin, the discoverer of PSA, certainly thinks it should and has been saying as much for years. Writing in 2010, he commented 'I never dreamed that my discovery four decades ago would lead to such a profit-driven public health disaster. The medical community must confront reality and stop the inappropriate use of PSA screening. Doing so would save billions of dollars and rescue millions of men from unnecessary, debilitating treatments'. At the very least, any man, before undergoing PSA testing, should be informed of the test's limitations and possible adverse consequences. As one group of experts noted: '[men] should be advised that the test cannot tell [them] whether they have a life-threatening cancer but that it could lead them through a thicket of tests and treatments that they might have better avoided'.[18]

Lung cancer screening: early but not early enough?

Screening may detect disease earlier, but not always early enough to make a difference (see Figure).

Some cancers, for example lung cancer, spread within the body before the patient has any symptoms and before any tests can detect the presence of the cancer. Attempts to detect lung cancer by the use of chest X-rays illustrate this problem (See stage B in Figure). In the 1970s, several large studies in heavy smokers

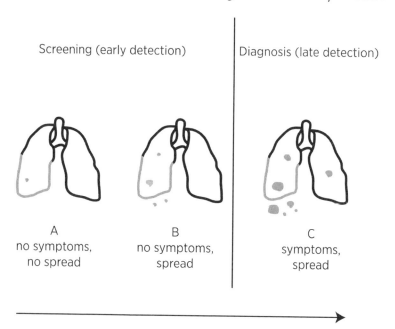

Growth and spread of lung cancer in heavy smokers.

SELLING SCREENING

'Selling screening can be easy. Induce fear by exaggerating risk. Offer hope by exaggerating the benefit of screening. And don't mention harms. It is especially easy with cancer — no diagnosis is more dreaded. And we all know the mantra: early detection is the best protection. Doubt it, and someone may suggest you need your head examined.

"If you are a woman over 35, be sure to schedule a mammogram. Unless you're still not convinced of its importance. In which case, you may need more than your breasts examined." Old American Cancer Society Poster.

Messages selling screening are everywhere. The news regularly tells the story of celebrities asserting that their lives have been saved because of the early diagnosis of a cancer. It is very unusual to hear stories of those injured by overdiagnosis and overtreatment.

Popular magazines report emotionally charged but wholly unrepresentative stories about young women with breast cancer and their fears of dying and leaving their young children.

Medical centers use screening as a business strategy, offering free tests to attract patients. Public service announcements — like the American Cancer Society's slogan above — speak for themselves.'

Woloshin S, Schwartz LM. Numbers needed to decide.
Journal of the National Cancer Institute 2009;101:1163-65.

showed that, although the cancers were detected earlier, there was no evidence this led to a decrease in deaths from the disease. The lung cancers detected on the X-rays had already spread beyond the lungs. So, these patients lived longer with their cancer diagnosis and were treated earlier, but there was no evidence that it made any difference to their life expectancy.

More recently, a large randomized trial involving 53,000 current and former heavy smokers compared chest X-ray screening with screening by a special sort of computed tomography (CT) scan called a spiral CT. Both groups were assigned to three annual screening procedures. Spiral CT diagnosed lung cancers at an even earlier stage than did chest X-rays, and in a small proportion of patients this was sufficiently early (stage A in Figure) for treatment to be of benefit (346 deaths from lung cancer in the spiral CT group vs 425 in the chest X-ray group). But this beneficial outcome came at the expense of a large proportion of people wrongly labelled with lung cancer. Overall, for every 1,000 heavy smokers who had three annual X-rays or scans, over eight years of follow-up, three fewer died of lung cancer. But 13 still died of lung cancer despite earlier detection, and 233 received a false-positive result that required further investigation.[19]

Genetic tests: sometimes useful, often dodgy

Not so long ago 'genetic testing' was more or less confined to generally rare, single-gene disorders – for example, the childhood-onset muscle-wasting disease Duchenne muscular dystrophy, or Huntington's disease, a progressive nervous system disorder that usually starts to affect people in middle age. Genetic tests are done to diagnose such conditions but can also be used to screen healthy people whose family history indicates that their chances of developing the disorder in question are above average, and to guide their family plans.

However, most diseases cannot be attributed to a single faulty gene. Usually, diseases depend on the way in which risk variants in several genes interact, and on the interaction of these genetic risk variants with environmental factors. Only when there is a 'critical' combination of genetic risk variants and environmental factors will a disease become apparent.[1]

Despite the complexity of ascribing most conditions to aberrant genes, media and promoters of direct-to-consumer genetic testing extol the supposed virtue and simplicity of genetic risk profiling. All you need to do is send off a saliva sample to a company for DNA analysis and they will take your money and send you your profile. But the information you receive is unlikely to help you – or your clinician – make any sensible predictions

DON'T PLAY POKER WITH YOUR GENES

'Acting on the knowledge of a single (or even a few) gene variants is similar to betting all your money on a poker hand when you've only seen one card. You don't know what hand genetic factors has dealt you, nor what effects your environment will have, and here, instead of 5 cards, there are over 20,000 genes and many thousands of environmental factors. And the effect of one gene may be cancelled out by the effect of lifestyle, family history or by the presence of other, protective genes. Many of us carry faulty genes without them ever causing disease.'

Sense About Science. *Making sense of testing: a guide to why scans and other health tests for well people aren't always a good idea.* London: Sense About Science 2008, p7. Available from www.senseaboutscience.org

about your risk of disease, let alone what might be done about it, if anything. This 'do-it-yourself' approach clearly does not meet the criteria for a useful screening test (see below). However, the result may well make you anxious and decision-making difficult, and may have wider implications too – on members of your family, for example. As one Australian health journalist put it 'For anyone concerned about the creeping medicalisation of life, the marketplace for genetic testing is surely one of the latest frontiers, where apparently harmless technology can help mutate healthy people into fearful patients, their personhood redefined by multiple genetic predispositions for disease and early death.'[20]

What screening aims to achieve and why evidence matters
The examples we have already given show that, before rushing headlong into widespread screening, it is worth pausing a moment to consider the key features of screening programmes and to remind ourselves what they aim to achieve. People being offered screening do not have, or have not noticed, the symptoms or signs of the condition being tested for – they have not sought medical attention for the disorder in question. The purpose of screening

individuals or populations is to reduce the risk of death or future ill health from a specific condition by offering a test intended to help identify people who could benefit from treatment.[1, 21] The aim of screening is not simply to diagnose disease earlier – this may not help anyone and it can even do harm.

The basic criteria for assessing the value of screening tests were outlined in a World Health Organization report in 1968.[22] These criteria have been further refined to reflect the way in which healthcare is delivered today. People invited for screening need sufficient, balanced information about the test being offered – including possible harms, consequences, and limitations, as well as potential benefits – so that they can make an informed choice. Essentially, the key points can be summed up by saying don't screen unless:

- The condition being screened for is important in terms of public health – for example, it is serious and/or affects large numbers of people
- There is a recognizable early stage of the condition
- There is an effective and acceptable treatment for the condition, so screening is likely to make a difference to its outcome
- There is a valid and reliable test for the condition that is acceptable to people being offered screening
- The screening programme is of good quality and cost-effective in the setting in which it is to be offered
- The information provided to people is unbiased; based on good evidence; and clear about possible harms (eg, overdiagnosis leading to over-treatment) as well as potential benefits
- The invitation for screening is not coercive – that is, it indicates it is reasonable to decline
- The chance of physical or psychological harm to those offered screening is likely to be less than the chance of benefit
- There are adequate facilities for the diagnosis and treatment of abnormalities detected by screening

THE SCREENING CIRCUS

In 2009, a recently retired professor of neurology with a long-standing interest in stroke prevention learnt that neighbours had received a leafleted invitation to be screened for stroke and other complications of cardiovascular disease. The leaflet, from a vascular screening company, invited them to go along to a local church (and pay £152, $230, €170) for a series of tests. Intrigued – not least because some of the information in the leaflet was factually misleading – he decided to go along himself.

'First up was aortic aneurysm [enlargement of the main artery carrying blood from the heart] screening with ultrasonography done by a woman who did not want to be engaged in conversation about what the implications of finding an aneurysm might be. Next it was ankle and arm blood pressure measurements "for troubles with my circulation" . . . followed by a little non-vascular bonus: osteoporosis screening of my ankle. Then there was . . . electrocardiography to detect "trouble with the two upper chambers of my heart" . . . Then, finally, carotid [artery in the neck] ultrasonography to detect "plaque build up". When I asked them what the implications of this might be they told me that blood clots could form and cause a stroke. Pressed on the sort of treatment I might be given, they offered a vague notion of blood thinning drugs but nothing about surgery until I asked directly if that might be an option, and indeed it was. "Might that be risky?" I enquired innocently. The answer was that any risks would depend on a full work-up by my GP, with whom I should discuss abnormalities from any of the tests.

All of this was conducted without any privacy (except for the aortic aneurysm screening) . . . There seemed to be no doctor present, and the team showed no intention or will to engage in a discussion of the implications of false positive or false negative results, the prognostic implications of true abnormalities, or the risks and benefits of any treatments.

This was just screening, nothing more and nothing less, done for profit – with the results to be dumped in my lap within 21 working days and for my GP to sort out the emotional and physical consequences of any abnormality, true or false, even though she didn't request the tests. . . . Inevitably this whole screening circus is liable to whip up anxiety in vulnerable people without discussing or taking the slightest responsibility for the consequences of any abnormalities found.'

Warlow C. The new religion: screening at your parish church. *BMJ* 2009;338:b1940

These criteria reinforce our message at the beginning of this chapter: that any decision to introduce a screening programme should be based on good-quality evidence not only about its effectiveness but also about its potential for doing harm.

IS ANYONE NORMAL?

Whole-body CT scans

Among the tests on offer at private clinics are whole-body computed tomography (CT) scans to look at head, neck, chest, abdomen, and pelvis. They are offered directly to the public, and usually done without reference to the person's general/primary care practitioner. Whole-body scans are often promoted as the way to keep one step ahead of possible illness, with the premise that a 'normal' result will be reassuring. Not only are these scans expensive, but also there is no evidence that any overall health benefit is achieved by doing these tests in people without symptoms or signs of disease.

Moreover, the radiation exposure is considerable – as much as 400 times more than a chest X-ray. So much so that in 2007 the UK's Committee on Medical Aspects of Radiation in the Environment (COMARE) strongly recommended that 'services' offering whole-body CT screening of asymptomatic individuals should discontinue to do so.

In 2010, after consultation, the Government announced its intention to introduce tougher rules for using whole-body scans. Similarly, the US Food and Drug Administration has warned the public that these scans have no proven benefits for healthy people, commenting 'Many people don't realize that getting a whole body CT screening exam won't necessarily give them the "peace of mind" that they are hoping for, or the information that would allow them to prevent a health problem. An abnormal finding, for example, may not be a serious one, and a normal finding may be inaccurate.' [23, 24, 25]

Striking a balance

Striking a balance between over-zealous trawling for disease and failing to identify those people who may benefit from early detection is never going to be easy, and will inevitably lead to unpopular decisions. All healthcare systems need to use their resources thriftily if the whole population is to benefit. This fundamental principle surely means that screening programmes must not only be based on sound evidence when they are introduced but also kept under review to check whether they are helpful as more evidence accrues and circumstances change. A serious consideration is whether screening programmes should be offered to large sectors of the population or more targeted towards those at high risk of a condition.

KEY POINTS

- Earlier diagnosis does not necessarily lead to better outcomes; sometimes it makes matters worse

- Screening programmes should only be introduced on the basis of sound evidence about their effects

- Not introducing a screening programme can be the best choice

- People invited for screening need balanced information

- The benefits of screening are often oversold

- The harms of screening are often downplayed or ignored

- Good communication about the benefits, harms, and risks of screening is essential

5 Dealing with uncertainty about the effects of treatments

In this chapter we look at the uncertainties that almost invariably surround the claimed effects of treatments, whether new or old. For example, few would probably question the routine use of oxygen in people who have had a heart attack, yet there is no good evidence that it helps, and some evidence that it may cause harm. This uncertainty has never been adequately addressed[1] and many other effects of treatments are disputed.

DRAMATIC TREATMENT EFFECTS: RARE AND READILY RECOGNIZABLE

Only rarely will the evidence be so clear-cut that there is no room for doubt about whether a treatment works.[2] In such cases the treatment effect is often dramatic and immediate. Take the heart rhythm disorder known as ventricular fibrillation, where muscle contraction in the ventricles (lower chambers) of the heart becomes wildly uncoordinated. This is a medical emergency – death can occur in minutes. The technique of 'zapping' the heart with a direct electrical current from a defibrillator applied to the chest is used to restore the heart's normal rhythm; when successful, the effect is virtually instantaneous.

Other dramatic effects (see also Chapter 6, p70) include drainage of pus to relieve pain from abscesses, blood transfusion for shock caused by severe haemorrhage, and insulin (a hormone produced by the pancreas) for diabetes. Up to the 1920s, patients with diabetes had short lives and suffered immensely, wasting away with uncontrollably high blood sugar levels. Very quickly, the initial results of animal tests led to the use of insulin in patients, with outstanding success – their response was near miraculous at the time. Another example from that era was the use of liver – later shown to be a source of vitamin B12 – for patients with pernicious anaemia. In this then fatal type of anaemia, the numbers of red blood cells gradually fall to disastrously low levels, leaving patients with a ghostly pallor and profound weakness. When these patients were given liver extract they recovered rapidly, and vitamin B12 is now prescribed routinely for this form of anaemia.

Some examples from the beginning of this century highlight similarly dramatic results.

Laser treatment of portwine stains

The birthmarks known as portwine stains are caused by permanent and malformed dilated blood vessels in the skin. Commonly occurring on the face, they persist and often darken as the child matures, and can be seriously disfiguring. Numerous treatments were tried over the years including freezing, surgery, and radiation, but with little impact and many side-effects. The introduction of laser treatment brought impressive results: improvement is usually seen after a single laser session in most types of lesions, and the damage caused by dispersion of heat from the laser to the surrounding skin tissues is temporary.[2, 3]

Imatinib for chronic myeloid leukaemia

Impressive results have also been seen in patients given imatinib for chronic myeloid leukaemia.[4, 5]

Before imatinib was introduced in the late 1990s, this type of leukaemia responded very poorly to standard treatments. When the new drug was tried, initially in patients who had not responded to standard therapy, the outlook for patients improved greatly. Imatinib stabilizes the disease, appears to prolong life substantially by comparison with the pre-imatinib era, and has mostly mild side-effects. It is now regarded as the first treatment option.

Mother's kiss

Low-tech approaches can have dramatic effects too. Young children sometimes place small objects – plastic toys or beads, for example – in their nose. But they often have trouble blowing their nose to expel such foreign bodies. The 'mother's kiss' technique for dislodging the offending object – involving a parent closing the unblocked nostril while blowing into the child's mouth – is simplicity itself, as well as being very effective.[2, 6]

A new treatment for strawberry birthmarks

Treatments with dramatic effects are occasionally discovered by accident. Take the example of a condition that occurs in infants called a haemangioma, which, like portwine stains, is also due to malformation of immature blood vessels. In haemangiomas, small blood vessels come together to form a lump. Haemangiomas mostly affect the skin, usually on the head and neck, but they can occur in organs inside the body such as the liver. The skin lesions, which are often called strawberry marks because of their bright red, raised appearance, are not usually visible at birth but generally appear in the first week or so of life. They tend to grow rapidly in the first three months and then the growth rate slows. In most cases they disappear of their own accord by the time the child is five years old, leaving behind a faint pink mark or some loose skin.

However, some haemangiomas need treatment because of their position – for example, they may cover an eye or block the nose. Or treatment may be necessary because of other complications. Ulcerated haemangiomas may become infected, or heart failure may develop in patients with very large lesions because the heart has to pump so much blood through blood vessels in the lump.

Until recently, steroids were the first-choice medical treatment for problematic haemangiomas. Then in 2008, some doctors had dramatic results with another treatment, which they came across quite by chance. They were using steroids to treat a baby with a huge haemangioma that almost swallowed up the face and right eye. Despite this treatment, however, the baby developed heart failure. So, to treat the heart failure they started the baby on a standard drug for this condition called propranolol. To their astonishment, the appearance of the haemangioma started

STEPWISE PROGRESS DOESN'T HIT THE HEADLINES

'Science itself works very badly as a news story: it is by its very nature a subject for the "features" section, because it does not generally move ahead by sudden, epoch-making breakthroughs. It moves ahead by gradually emergent themes and theories, supported by a raft of evidence from a number of different disciplines on a number of different explanatory levels. Yet the media remain obsessed with "new breakthroughs".'

Goldacre B. *Bad Science*. London: Fourth Estate, 2008, p219.

to improve within 24 hours, and within a week the tumour had shrunk sufficiently for the baby to open an eyelid. After six months of treatment the haemangioma had melted away. Over the following year the doctors went on to use propranolol in a dozen children with similar success. These impressive results have been replicated by other doctors in small numbers of children and propranolol is now being studied further in larger numbers of infants.[7,8]

MODERATE TREATMENT EFFECTS: USUAL AND NOT SO OBVIOUS

Most treatments do not have dramatic effects and fair tests are needed to assess them. And sometimes a treatment may have a dramatic effect in some circumstances but not in others.

Although vitamin B12 is undoubtedly effective for pernicious anaemia (see above), dispute continues to this day about whether patients need quarterly or more frequent treatment. That question will only be answered by carefully controlled tests comparing the options. Moreover, whereas the pain relief with hip replacements is dramatic, the relative merits of different types of artificial hip joints are far more subtle, but may nevertheless be important – some may wear out faster than others for example. With laser treatment of portwine birthmarks (see above), there is also still much to learn. Whilst this treatment remains the 'gold standard', research continues into why some lesions re-darken after several years, and on the effects of different types of lasers, possibly combined with cooling of the skin.[9, 10]

And while aspirin substantially reduces the risk of death in patients suffering a heart attack if given promptly on diagnosis, whether taking aspirin to prevent heart attacks and strokes does more harm than good depends on whether patients have underlying cardiovascular disease. The benefits – reduction in the risk of heart attacks, strokes, and death from cardiovascular causes – need to be balanced against the risks – bleeding, especially the type of stroke caused by bleeding into the brain, and bleeding from the gut. In patients who already have cardiovascular disease, the benefits of the drug greatly outweigh the risks. But in otherwise healthy people, the benefits of aspirin do not clearly outweigh the risk of bleeding (see Chapter 7).[11]

WHEN PRACTITIONERS DISAGREE

For many diseases and conditions, there is substantial uncertainty about the extent to which treatments work, or about which treatment is best for which patient. That doesn't stop some doctors having very strong opinions about treatments, even though those opinions may differ from one doctor to the next. This can lead to considerable variation in the treatments prescribed for a given condition.

In the 1990s, Iain Chalmers, one of the authors, while holidaying in the USA, broke an ankle and was treated by an orthopaedic surgeon. The surgeon put the leg in a temporary splint, and said that the next step, once the swelling had subsided, would be a lower leg plaster cast for six weeks. On returning home a couple of days later, Iain went to the local fracture clinic, where a British orthopaedic surgeon, without hesitation, dismissed this advice. Putting the leg in plaster, the British surgeon said, would be wholly inappropriate. In the light of this obvious professional uncertainty, Iain asked whether he could participate in a controlled comparison to find out which treatment was better.

The British surgeon answered that controlled trials are for people who are uncertain whether or not they are right – and that he was certain that he was right.

How can such a pronounced difference in professional opinion come about, and what is a patient to make of this? Each surgeon was certain, individually, about the correct course of action. Yet their widely divergent views clearly revealed uncertainty within the profession as a whole about the best way to treat a common fracture. Was there good evidence about which treatment was better? If so, was one or neither surgeon aware of the evidence? Or was it that nobody knew which treatment was better (see Figure).

Perhaps the two surgeons differed in the value they placed on particular outcomes of treatments: the American surgeon may have been more concerned about relief of pain – hence the recommendation of a plaster cast – while his British counterpart may have been more worried about the possibility of muscle wasting, which occurs when a limb is immobilized in this way. If so, why did neither surgeon ask Iain which outcome mattered more to him, the patient? Two decades later, uncertainty continues about how to manage this very common condition.[12]

There are several separate issues here. First, was there any reliable evidence comparing the two very different approaches being recommended? If so, did the evidence show their relative effects on outcomes (reduced pain, or reduced muscle wasting, for example) that might matter to Iain or to other patients, who might have different preferences to his? But what if there was no evidence providing the information needed?

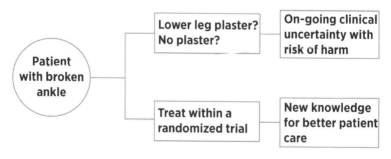

What should a doctor do?

FACING UP TO UNCERTAINTIES:
A MATTER OF LIFE AND DEATH

'Failure to face up to uncertainties about the effects of treatments can result in avoidable suffering and death on a massive scale. If when diazepam and phenytoin were introduced as anticonvulsants for eclampsia they had been compared with magnesium sulphate – which had been in use for decades – hundreds of thousands fewer women would have suffered and died. Similarly, if the effects of systemic steroids for traumatic brain injury had been assessed before this treatment became widely adopted, tens of thousands of unnecessary deaths could have been avoided. These are just two examples of many that might have been used to illustrate why doctors have a professional responsibility to help address uncertainties about the effects of treatments.'

Chalmers I. Addressing uncertainties about the effects of treatments offered to NHS patients: whose responsibility? *Journal of the Royal Society of Medicine* 2007; 100: 440.

Some clinicians are clear about what to do when there is no reliable evidence about the effects of alternative treatments and are prepared to discuss this uncertainty with patients. For example, one doctor who specializes in caring for people with stroke, commented that, although research evidence shows that his patients would fare better if cared for in a stroke unit, it remained uncertain – for many types of patients – whether they should receive clot-busting drugs (see also Chapter 11, p139). When discussing treatment options with his patients he explained that these drugs may do more good than harm, but they may – for some patients – actually do more harm than good. He then went on to explain why, talking to a patient for whom the balance of risk and benefit was unclear, he felt he could only recommend this treatment for them within the context of a carefully controlled comparison, which should help to reduce the uncertainty.[13] Uncertainties about several aspects of clot-busting drugs persist.[14]

ADDRESSING UNCERTAINTY IS PROFESSIONAL

'One of the key attributes of professionalism . . . should be the ability to identify and address uncertainty in medicine. Every day professionals confront and cope with uncertainties about disease pathogenesis, about diagnosis, and about treatment. Yet the intrinsic uncertainties in all these spheres of medical activity are seldom acknowledged explicitly and some professionals remain uncomfortable about admissions of uncertainty – in their dealings with patients especially. Uncertainty is also a prime stimulus for medical research to improve human health, which is central to the MRC's mission. In the future it will be increasingly important for medical professionals to take on board the results of accumulated research findings relevant to their area of practice so that they are aware where continuing uncertainties exist and what research is ongoing or needed to address these. Overall, a mark of professionalism for the future will be research awareness for the benefit of patients. Some medical professionals will actively participate in research but all should seek to encourage it and, where appropriate, to involve their patients actively in the medical research agenda, and implement the results of this research in their professional practice.'

From: Medical Research Council response to Royal College of Physicians consultation on medical professionalism. 2005

Caffeine for breathing problems in premature babies

Large variations in the treatments used for a particular condition provide clear evidence of professional uncertainty about the relative merits of different treatments. And entrenched practices may mean that it takes a very long time for such uncertainties to be addressed by fair tests. The use of caffeine in premature babies provides a telling example. Such babies often have trouble breathing properly and sometimes stop breathing very briefly – this condition is known as apnoea of prematurity and affects most babies born at less than 34 weeks' gestation. In the late 1970s, caffeine treatment was shown to reduce these episodes and then became used by some paediatricians.

However the effects of caffeine remained disputed. Although fair tests had shown that caffeine reduced the episodes of apnoea, many paediatricians did not think that the episodes were sufficiently serious to justify use of the drug, and some were concerned that it might not be safe in these tiny babies. This meant that some babies were given the treatment and others weren't. When these widespread uncertainties were finally assessed by a large international study more than 30 years after the treatment had been introduced, it turned out that this simple therapy not only reduces the breathing difficulties but also, and very importantly, significantly improves the likelihood of long-term survival without cerebral palsy and delay in infant development. Had this uncertainty been addressed when the treatment was introduced, fewer babies would have gone on to develop disabilities.[15, 16]

Antibiotics in pre-term labour

Fair tests of treatments with hoped-for beneficial effects, and which are assumed to be harmless, can show that neither is true. Doctors prescribe treatments with the best of intentions, particularly when they may offer hope in a desperate situation. For example, a theory suggested that 'silent' (sub-clinical) infection might trigger early labour and preterm delivery. The theory led doctors to prescribe antibiotics for some pregnant women in the hope that this might help to prolong pregnancy. No one seriously thought that using antibiotics in this way would cause any serious problems. Indeed, there is some evidence that women themselves were keen to have antibiotics – in a spirit of 'let's try this; it can't do any harm'.

When a fair test of this treatment was eventually done, the results had clear clinical implications. For a start, no benefits were identified. On top of that, long-term follow-up of the babies in the study showed that those who had been exposed to antibiotics were more likely than those in the comparison groups to have cerebral palsy and problems with speech, vision, and walking. These risks of antibiotics had remained unrecognized over the decades that

DOCTORS TALKING ABOUT GUESSWORK IN PRESCRIBING

In a fictional conversation between two doctors, a general practitioner makes the following point: 'Tons of what we do is guesswork and I don't think that you or I feel too comfortable with that. The only way to find out if something works is a proper trial, but the hoops are huge. So what do we do? We do what we fancy. And I'm sure some of the time it's fine – clinical experience and all that. Maybe the rest of the time we're just as likely to be getting it wrong as right, but because whatever we're doing isn't called a trial, no one regulates it and none of us learn from it'.

Adapted from Petit-Zeman S. Doctor, what's wrong?
Making the NHS human again. London: Routledge, 2005, pp79-80.

antibiotics had been prescribed to women, but without adequate evidence from fair tests about their effects. As often happens, those who were given an inadequately evaluated treatment in 'normal' clinical practice were more likely to be harmed than those given the same treatment prescribed in a research context. Put another way, people were generally more at risk when they were not taking the drugs as part of a fair test.[17, 18, 19]

Breast cancer

The treatment of breast cancer (see Chapter 3) provides another example of professional uncertainty. There is considerable variability in the use of surgery, radiotherapy, and chemotherapy. The best treatment of very early stage breast cancers and of 'pseudo-cancers' of the breast is unresolved, as is the ideal number of lymph nodes to remove from the armpit, or indeed whether any should be removed at all.[20] As if that were not enough, topics of particular interest to patients, such as relief of fatigue associated with therapy, or the best way of treating lymphoedema of the arm – a distressing and disabling aftermath of surgery and radiotherapy in the armpit – still have not been tested adequately.

ADDRESSING UNCERTAINTIES ABOUT THE EFFECTS OF TREATMENTS

Where do we go from here? Clinicians need to be able to draw on resources that provide the best current evidence about a treatment, taken from collective experience and systematic reviews of any reliable research studies that exist. If, after doing this, they find that uncertainty remains about a treatment, they need to be prepared to discuss this with their patients and to explain why this is so. Patients and clinicians can then discuss the options together, taking into account patient preferences. These discussions may raise further uncertainties that need to be acknowledged and addressed. Only by recognizing together that uncertainties still exist, can steady progress be made towards making treatments more appropriate and safer. Uncertainty is therefore a prerequisite for progress, not an admission of 'defeat'. This positive attitude to addressing uncertainties is now reflected in some professional guidance. In the UK, the General Medical Council's latest version of its *Good Medical Practice* guidance instructs doctors that, as part of maintaining and improving their performance, they 'must help to resolve uncertainties about the effects of treatments'.[21] To do this, patients and clinicians must work together to design better research (see Chapter 11).

PROVIDING TREATMENT AS PART OF A FAIR TEST

So what should happen when there is important uncertainty about the effects of new or old treatments that have not been properly evaluated? An obvious answer is to follow the example of the doctor caring for his stroke patients, as we described above: address the uncertainty by offering inadequately assessed treatments only within the context of research that has been designed to find out more about both their wanted and unwanted effects.

A medical ethicist put it this way:

'If we are uncertain about the relative intrinsic merits of any [different] treatments, then we cannot be certain about those merits in any given use of one of them – as in treating an individual patient. So it seems irrational and unethical to insist one way or another before completion of a suitable trial. Thus the answer to the question, "What is the best treatment for the patient?" is: "The trial". The trial is the treatment. Is this experimentation? Yes. But all we mean by that is choice under uncertainty, plus data collection. Does it matter that the choice is "random"? Logically, no. After all, what better mechanism is there for choice under uncertainty?'[22]

Providing treatments as part of fair tests can help to make a profound difference to outcomes for patients. The story of childhood leukaemia provides a very dramatic example of this. Until the 1960s, virtually every child with leukaemia died soon after the diagnosis had been made. Now about 85 children out of 100 survive. This has been achieved because most children with leukaemia have participated in randomized trials comparing the current standard treatment with a new variant of that treatment.[23] For most children with cancer, therefore, the best treatment

---

CAN PATIENTS COPE WITH UNCERTAINTY?

'So where are we with addressing uncertainties about the effects of treatments? . . . Despite general acknowledgement that patients are partners in medical research and healthcare decisions, the complexity of discussing therapeutic uncertainty is unnerving some doctors. Some are simply fearful of provoking anxiety – doubtless a genuine concern but nevertheless paternalistic. Others try to justify their actions in terms of a balance between two ethical arguments – whether the ethical duty to tell the truth extends to being explicit about uncertainties versus the moral obligation to protect patients from emotional burden. Are patients prepared to live with uncertainty? We need to find out. Perhaps people are far more resilient than doctors suspect.'

Evans I. More nearly certain. *Journal of the Royal Society of Medicine* 2005;98:195-6.

option is chosen by participation in such trials.

If no such trial is available, at the very least the results of using new and untested treatments should be recorded in a standardized way – for example, by using a checklist of items including the laboratory or other tests that will be used to diagnose a condition and the tests that will be done to assess the impact of the treatment. The plan of investigation could also be registered in a database, as should happen for clinical trials (see Chapter 8). By doing this, the results can contribute to the body of knowledge for the benefit of the patients receiving the untested treatment and patients everywhere. Huge sums of money have already been invested in healthcare IT systems, which could readily be used to capture this information for the benefit of patients and of the public (see also Chapter 11).[24]

There will have to be changes if uncertainties about the effects of treatments are to be addressed more effectively and efficiently. We discuss some of these – particularly the greater involvement of patients – later in the book (see Chapters 11 and 12). However, there is a particular issue – we touched on it above – that we want to emphasize here. When there is insufficient information about the effects of a treatment, knowledge can be increased by ensuring that clinicians only offer it within the context of a formal evaluation until more is known about its value and possible disadvantages. Yet some prevailing attitudes, including systems of research regulation (see Chapter 9), actually discourage this risk-limiting approach.

The problem vexed a British paediatrician over 30 years ago when he pithily observed that he needed permission to give a treatment to half his patients (that is, to find out about its effects by giving half the patients the new treatment and half the existing treatment in a controlled comparison), but not if he wanted to give the same treatment to all of them as a standard prescription.[25] This illogical double standard still pops up repeatedly and discourages clinicians who want to reduce uncertainties about the effects of their treatments. The overall effect is that health professionals can be deterred from generating knowledge from their experiences in treating patients. As the American sociologist Charles Bosk once remarked: 'anything goes, as long as we promise not to learn from the experience'.

Being able to explain uncertainty clearly demands skills and a certain degree of humility on the part of doctors. Many feel uneasy when trying to explain to potential participants in a clinical trial that no one knows which treatment is best. But the public's attitude has changed: arrogant doctors who 'play God' are increasingly given short shrift. We need to focus on training doctors who are not ashamed to admit they are human and that they need the help and the participation of patients in research to provide more certainty about choices of treatments (see Chapters 11 and 12).

The main stumbling block for many clinicians and patients is lack of familiarity with the features of fair tests of treatments, an issue we tackle next (see Chapter 6).

KEY POINTS

- Dramatic effects of treatments are rare

- Uncertainties about the effects of treatments are very common

- Small differences in the effects of different treatments are usual, and it is important to detect these reliably

- When nobody knows the answer to an important uncertainty about the effects of a treatment, steps need to be taken to reduce the uncertainty

- Much more could be done to help patients contribute to reducing uncertainties about the effects of treatments

---

6 Fair tests of treatments

The principles underlying fair tests of treatments may not be familiar to many readers, but they are not complicated. In fact, much of our everyday, intuitive grasp of the world depends on them. Yet they are not taught well in schools and are often needlessly wrapped up in complex language. As a result, many people shy away from the subject, believing that it is beyond their ability to comprehend. We hope this and the following two chapters will persuade you that you are actually already aware of the key principles, and so will readily understand why they are so important. Readers who would like to explore these issues in more detail will find additional material at www.testingtreatments.org and in *The James Lind Library* (www.jameslindlibrary.org).

WHY ARE FAIR TESTS OF TREATMENTS NEEDED?

Nature, the healer

Many health problems will tend to get worse without treatment, and some will get worse in spite of treatment. However, some get better by themselves – that is, they are 'self-limiting'. As one researcher involved in testing a proposed treatment for the common cold put it: 'if a cold is treated energetically it will get well in seven days, while if left to itself it will get well in a week'.[1] Put more cynically, 'Nature cures, but the doctor takes the fee.'

And of course, treatment may actually make matters worse.

It is because people often recover from illness without any specific treatment that the 'natural' progress and outcome of illnesses without treatment must be taken into account when treatments are being tested. Think about a time when you have had a sore throat, a stomach cramp, or an unusual skin rash. These will often resolve on their own, without formal treatment. Yet, if you *had* received treatment (even an ineffective treatment), you might have assumed that the treatment caused the symptoms to disappear. In short, knowledge of the natural history of an illness, including the likelihood that it will get better on its own (spontaneous remission), can prevent use of un-needed treatments and false beliefs in unproven remedies.

When symptoms of an illness come and go, it is especially difficult to try to pin down the effects of treatments. Patients with arthritis, for example, are most likely to seek help when they are having a particularly bad flare-up – which, by its very nature, is unlikely to be sustained. Whether the treatment they then receive is mainstream or complementary, effective or ineffective, it is

---

MISTAKING THE CURE

. . .'it is alleged to be found true by proof, that by the taking of *Tobacco,* divers and very many do find themselves cured of divers diseases; as on the other part, no man ever received harm thereby. In this argument there is first a great mistaking, and next a monstrous absurdity: . . .when a sick man has his disease at the height, he hath at that instant taken *Tobacco,* and afterward his disease taking the natural course of declining and consequently the patient of recovering his health, O then the *Tobacco* forsooth, was the worker of that miracle.'

James Stuart, King of Great Britaine, France and Ireland. A counterblaste to tobacco. In: *The workes of the most high and mightie prince, James.* Published by James, Bishop of Winton, and Deane of his Majesties Chappel Royall. London: printed by Robert Barker and John Bill, printers to the Kings most excellent Majestie, 1616: pp 214-222.

likely that their pain will improve after receiving it, simply because the flare-up dies down. Understandably, however, practitioners and patients will tend to attribute such improvements to the treatment taken, even though it may have had nothing to do with the improvements.

The beneficial effects of optimism and wishful thinking

The psychological reasons for people attributing any improvement in their condition to the treatment they received are now better understood. We all have a tendency to assume that if one event follows another, the first may have been responsible for the second. And we are inclined to see patterns where none exist – a phenomenon that has been demonstrated many times in areas as diverse as coin tossing, stock market prices and basketball shots. We are all also prone to a problem known as confirmation bias: we see what we expect to see – 'believing is seeing'. Any support we find for our beliefs will boost our confidence that we are right. Conversely, we may not recognize or readily accept information that contradicts our views, and so tend to turn a blind eye to it – often unconsciously.

BELIEVING IS SEEING

The British doctor Richard Asher noted in one of his essays for doctors:

'If you can believe fervently in your treatment, even though controlled tests show that it is quite useless, then your results are much better, your patients are much better, and your income is much better, too. I believe this accounts for the remarkable success of some of the less gifted, but more credulous members of our profession, and also for the violent dislike of statistics and controlled tests which fashionable and successful doctors are accustomed to display.'

Asher R. Talking sense (Lettsomian lecture, 16 Feb, 1959). *Transactions of the Medical Society of London*, vol LXXV, 1958-59. Reproduced in: Jones, FA, ed. *Richard Asher talking sense*. London: Pitman Medical, 1972.

Most patients and clinicians hope, of course, that treatments will help. They may conclude that something works simply because it agrees with their belief that it *should* work. They do not look for, or they discard, information that is contrary to their beliefs. These psychological effects also explain why patients who believe that a treatment will help to relieve their symptoms may well experience improvements in their condition – even though the treatment, in fact, has no active ingredient (a 'sham', often known as a 'placebo'). Patients have reported improvements after being given pills made of sugar, injections of water, treatments with inactivated electric gadgetry, and surgery where nothing happened other than a small cut being made and sewn up again.

Take the example of a test comparing different weight-reducing diets. Researchers recruited viewers of a popular television programme who wanted to lose weight and assigned them to one of six diets. One of the diets – *bai lin* tea – had been promoted as a successful way of losing weight. The average weight of the slimmers went down in all six groups, but in some much more than in others. However, when the results were presented on television, it was revealed that one of the diets – 'the carrot diet' – was not a slimming diet at all. It had been included in the test to provide a 'bench mark' of weight loss which was due not to any of the six diets, but to changes in eating habits resulting from other factors that had motivated participants to eat differently.[2]

The need to go beyond impressions

If patients believe that something helps them, isn't that enough? Why is it important to go to the trouble and expense of doing research to try to assess the effects of the treatment more formally, and perhaps to try to find out whether and if so *how* it has helped them? 'There are at least two reasons. One is that treatments that do not work may distract us from treatments that do work. Another reason is that many (if not most) treatments have adverse side-effects, some short term, some longer term, and some still unrecognized. If patients do not use these treatments, they can be spared the unwanted effects. So it is worth identifying treatments that are very unlikely to help or might cause more harm than benefit. Research may also uncover important information about how treatments work, and so indicate possibilities for developing better and safer treatments.

Research about the effects of treatments is relevant everywhere, but especially in communities that endeavour to share healthcare resources fairly among all patients – for example, in the British National Health Service, or the US Veterans Health Administration. In these circumstances, decisions always have to be taken about which treatments represent good value for the inevitably limited resources available for healthcare. If some patients are given treatments that have not been shown to be useful, this may mean depriving other patients of treatments that have been shown to be beneficial.

None of this should suggest that patients' and clinicians' impressions and ideas about the effects of treatments are unimportant. Indeed they are often the starting point for formal investigation of apparently promising new treatments. Following up such impressions with formal research can sometimes lead to the identification of both harmful and useful effects of treatments. For example, it was a woman who had been treated with the drug diethylstilboestrol (DES) during pregnancy two decades earlier who first suggested that this might have caused her daughter's rare vaginal cancer (see Chapter 2, p15-16). And when a patient mentioned unexpected side-effects of a new treatment prescribed for his raised blood pressure, neither he nor his doctor could have imagined that his comment would lead to the identification of an all-time best-selling drug – sildenafil (Viagra).

So, individuals' impressions about the effects of treatments should not be ignored, but they are seldom a reliable basis for drawing sound conclusions about the effects of treatments, let alone for recommending treatments to others.

So what are fair tests?

Most of us know that it can be a mistake to take a media report of some new medical advance at face value. But the sad truth is that one must also be cautious about reports of treatments even in apparently reputable journals. Misleading and overblown claims about treatments are common, and it is important to be able to assess their reliability.

We run two risks in taking reports of the effects of treatments at face value. We could wrongly conclude that a helpful treatment is actually useless or even dangerous. Or we could wrongly conclude that a useless or even dangerous treatment is actually helpful. Fair tests of treatments are designed to obtain reliable information about the effects of treatments by (i) comparing like with like, to reduce distorting influences (biases); (ii) taking account of the play of chance; and (iii) assessing all the relevant, reliable evidence. This chapter and the next two chapters deal with these three principal features of fair tests.

COMPARING LIKE WITH LIKE

Comparisons are key
Comparisons are key to all fair tests of treatments. Clinicians and patients sometimes compare in their minds the relative merits of two treatments. For example, they may form an impression that they or others are responding differently to a treatment compared with responses to previous treatments. Sometimes the comparisons are made more formally. As early as the ninth-century, the Persian physician al-Razi compared the outcome of patients with meningitis treated with blood-letting with the outcome of those treated without it to see if blood-letting could help.

Treatments are usually tested by comparing groups of patients who have received different treatments. If treatment comparisons are to be fair, the comparisons must ensure that like will be compared with like: that the only systematic difference between the groups of patients is the treatments they have received. This insight is not new. For example, before beginning his comparison of six treatments for scurvy on board HMS *Salisbury* in 1747, James Lind (i) took care to select patients who were at a similar stage of this often lethal disease; (ii) ensured that the patients had the same basic diet; and (iii) arranged for them to be accommodated in similar conditions (see Chapter 1, p1-3). Lind recognized that factors other than the treatments themselves might influence his patients' chances of recovery.

One way to make a test *unfair* would have been to give one of the treatments recommended for scurvy – say, sulphuric acid, which was being recommended by the Royal College of Physicians of London – to patients who were less ill to begin with and in the early stages of the disease, and another treatment – say, citrus fruits, which were being recommended by some sailors – to patients who were already approaching death. This would have made sulphuric acid appear to be better, even though it was actually worse. Biases such as these can arise unless care is taken to ensure that like is being compared with like in all relevant respects.

Treatments with dramatic effects

Sometimes patients experience responses to treatments which differ so dramatically from their own past experiences, and from the natural history of their illness, that confident conclusions about treatment effects can be drawn without carefully done tests (see Chapter 5, p50-53).[3] For a patient with a collapsed lung (pneumothorax), inserting a needle into the chest and letting out the trapped air causes such immediate relief that the benefits of this treatment are clear. Other examples of dramatic effects include morphine on pain, insulin in diabetic coma, and artificial hip joints on pain from arthritis. Adverse effects of treatment can be dramatic as well. Sometimes drugs provoke severe, even lethal, allergic reactions; other dramatic effects include the rare limb deformities caused by thalidomide (see Chapter 1, p4-5).

However, such dramatic effects of treatments, whether beneficial or harmful, are rare. Most treatment effects are more modest, but still worth knowing about. For example, carefully done tests are needed to identify which dosage schedules for morphine are effective and safe; or whether genetically engineered insulin has any advantages over animal insulins; or whether a newly marketed artificial hip that is 20 times more expensive than the least expensive variety is worth the extra cost in terms that patients can appreciate. In these common circumstances we all need to avoid unfair (biased) comparisons, and the mistaken conclusions that can result from them.

Treatments with moderate but important effects

Comparing patients given treatments today with apparently similar patients given other treatments in the past for the same disease
Researchers sometimes compare patients given treatments today with apparently similar patients given other treatments in the past for the same disease. Such comparisons can provide reliable evidence if the treatment effects are dramatic – for example, when a new treatment now leads some patients to survive from a disease that had been universally fatal. However, when the differences between the treatments are not dramatic, but nevertheless worth knowing about, such comparisons using 'historical controls' are potentially problematic. Although researchers use statistical adjustments and analyses to try to ensure that like will be compared with like, these analyses cannot take account of relevant features of patients in the comparison groups which have not been recorded. As a result, we can never be completely confident that like is being compared with like.

The problems can be illustrated by comparing the results of the same treatment given to similar patients, but at different points in time. Take an analysis of 19 such instances in patients with advanced lung cancer comparing the annual death rates experienced by similar patients treated at different points in time with exactly the same treatments. Although few differences in death rates would have been expected, in fact the differences were considerable: death rates ranged from 24% better to 46% worse.[4] Clearly, these differences were not because the treatments had changed – they were the same – or because the patients were detectably different – they weren't. The differing death rates presumably reflected either undetected differences between the patients, or other, unrecorded changes over time (better nursing or control of infection, for example), which could not be taken into account in the comparisons.

Comparing apparently similar groups of patients who happen to have received different treatments in the same time period
Comparing the experiences and outcomes of apparently similar groups of patients who happen to have received different treatments

in the same time period is still used as a way to try to assess the effects of treatments. However, this approach too can be seriously misleading. The challenge, as with comparisons using 'historical controls', is to know whether the groups of people receiving the different treatments were sufficiently alike before they started treatment for a valid comparison to be possible – in other words, whether like was being compared with like. As with 'historical controls', researchers may use statistical adjustments and analyses to try to ensure that like will be compared with like, but only if relevant features of patients in the comparison groups have been recorded and taken into account. So seldom will these conditions have been met that such analyses should always be viewed with great caution. Belief in them can lead to major tragedies.

A telling example concerns hormone replacement therapy (HRT). Women who had used HRT during and after the menopause were compared with apparently similar women who had not used it. These comparisons suggested that HRT reduced the risk of heart attacks and stroke – which would have been very welcome news if it were true. Unfortunately it wasn't. Subsequent comparisons, which were designed before treatment started to ensure that the comparison groups would be alike, showed that HRT had exactly the opposite effect – it actually increased heart attacks and strokes (see Chapter 2, p16-18). In this case, the apparent difference in the rates of heart attacks and strokes was due to the fact that the women who used HRT were generally healthier than those who did not take HRT – it was not due to the HRT. Research that has not ensured that like really is being compared with like can result in harm being done to tens of thousands of people.

As the HRT experience indicates, the best way to ensure that like will be compared with like is to assemble the comparison groups before starting treatment. The groups need to be composed of patients who are similar not just in terms of known and measured factors, such as age and the severity of their illness, but also in terms of unmeasured factors that may influence recovery from illness, such as diet, occupation and other social factors, or anxiety about illness or proposed treatments. It is always difficult – indeed often impossible – to be confident that treatment groups are alike if they have been assembled after treatment has started.

The critical question then is this: do differences in outcomes reflect differences in the effects of the *treatments* being compared, or differences in the *patients* in the comparison groups?

Unbiased, prospective allocation to different treatments

In 1854, Thomas Graham Balfour, an army doctor in charge of a military orphanage, showed how treatment groups could be created to ensure that like would be compared with like. Balfour wanted to find out whether belladonna protected children from scarlet fever, as some people were claiming. So, 'to avoid the imputation of selection' as he put it, he allocated children *alternately* either to receive the drug, or not to receive it.[5] The use of alternate allocation, or some other unbiased way of creating comparison groups, is a key feature of fair tests of treatments. It increases the likelihood that comparison groups will be similar, not just in terms of known and measured important factors, but also of unmeasured factors that may influence recovery from illness, and for which it is impossible to make statistical adjustments.

To achieve fair (unbiased) allocation to different treatments it is important that those who design fair tests ensure that clinicians and patients cannot know or predict what the next allocation will be. If they do know, they may be tempted, consciously or unconsciously, to choose particular treatments. For example, if a doctor knows that the next patient scheduled to join a clinical trial is due to get a placebo (a sham treatment), she or he might discourage a more seriously ill patient from joining the trial and wait for a patient who was less ill. So even if an unbiased allocation *schedule* has been produced, unbiased *allocation* to treatment groups will only occur if upcoming allocations in the schedule are successfully concealed from those taking decisions about whether or not a patient will join a trial. In this way, no one will be able to tell which treatment is going to be allocated next, and tempted to depart from the unbiased allocation schedule.

Allocation concealment is usually done by generating allocation schedules that are less predictable than simple alternation – for example, by basing allocation on random numbers – and by concealing the schedule. Several methods are used to conceal allocation schedules. For example, random allocation can be assigned remotely – by telephone or computer – for a patient confirmed as eligible to participate in the study. Another way is to use a series of numbered envelopes, each containing an allocation – when a patient is eligible for a study, the next envelope in the series is opened to reveal what the allocation is. For this system to work, the envelopes have to be opaque so that doctors can't 'cheat' by holding the envelope up to the light to see the allocation inside.

This approach is recognized today as a key feature of fair tests of treatments. Studies in which random numbers are used to allocate treatments are known as 'randomized trials' (see box in Chapter 3, p26).

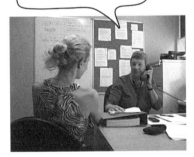
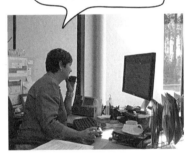

Concealing treatment allocation in a trial using telephone randomization.

Ways of using unbiased (random) allocation in treatment comparisons

Random allocation for treatment comparisons can be used in various ways. For example, it can be used to compare different treatments given at different times in random order to the same patient – a so-called 'randomized cross-over trial'. So, to assess whether an inhaled drug could help an individual patient with a persistent, dry cough, a study could be designed to last a few months. During some weeks, chosen randomly, the patient would use an inhaler containing a drug; during the other weeks the patient would use an identical-looking inhaler which did not contain the drug. Tailoring the results of research to individual patients in this way is clearly desirable if it can be done. But there are many circumstances in which such crossover studies are simply not possible. For example, different surgical operations cannot be compared in this way, and nor can treatments for 'one-off', acute health problems, such as severe bleeding after a road crash.

Random allocation can also be used to compare different treatments given to different parts of the same patient. So, in a skin disorder such as eczema or psoriasis, affected patches of skin can be selected at random to decide which should be treated with ointment containing a drug, and which with ointment without the active ingredients. Or in treating illness in both eyes, one of the eyes could be selected at random for treatment and comparison made with the untreated eye.

Another use of random allocation is to compare different treatments given to different populations or groups – say, all the people attending each of a number of primary care clinics

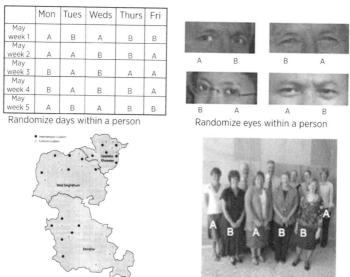

	Mon	Tues	Weds	Thurs	Fri
May week 1	A	B	A	B	B
May week 2	A	A	B	B	A
May week 3	B	A	B	A	A
May week 4	B	A	B	B	A
May week 5	A	B	A	B	B

Randomize days within a person

Randomize eyes within a person

Randomize communities within a region

Randomize individuals within a group

Different possible units for random allocation.

or hospitals. These comparisons are known as 'cluster (or group) randomized trials'. For example, to assess the effects of the Mexican universal health insurance programme, researchers matched 74 pairs of healthcare catchment areas – clusters that collectively represented 118,000 households in seven states. Within each matched pair one was allocated at random to the insurance programme.[6]

However by far the most common use of random allocation is its use to decide which patient will receive which treatment.

Following up everyone in treatment comparisons

After taking the trouble to assemble comparison groups to ensure that like will be compared with like, it is important to avoid introducing the bias that would result if the progress of some patients were to be ignored. As far as possible, all the patients allocated to the comparison groups should be followed up and included in the main analysis of the results of the group to which they were allocated, irrespective of which treatment (if any) they actually received. This is called an 'intention-to-treat' analysis. If this is not done, like will no longer be compared with like.

At first sight it may seem illogical to compare groups in which some patients have not received the treatments to which they were assigned, but ignoring this principle can make the tests unfair and the results misleading. For example, patients who have partial blockages of blood vessels supplying the brain and who experience dizzy spells are at above average risk of having a stroke. Researchers conducted a test to find out whether an operation to unclog blood vessels in these patients would reduce subsequent strokes. They rightly compared all the patients allocated to have the operation, irrespective of whether they survived the surgery, with all those allocated not to have it. If they had recorded the frequency of strokes only among patients who survived the immediate effects of the operation, they would have missed the important fact that the surgery itself can cause stroke and death and, other things being equal, the surviving patients in this group will have fewer strokes. That would have been an unfair test of the effects of the operation, the risks of which need to be factored into the assessment.

The outcomes of surgery and medical treatment shown in the

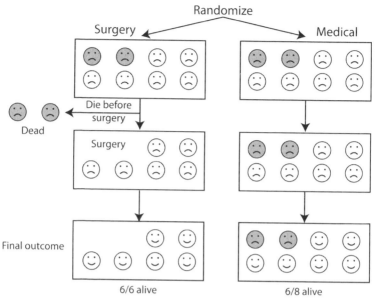

Why all patients randomized should be included in the final outcome ('intention to treat').

figure are actually equal. However, if the two people allocated to surgery die before operation and are then excluded from consideration, the comparison of the two groups will be biased. It will suggest that surgery appears to be better when it is not.

Dealing with departures from allocated treatments

For all the reasons given so far in this chapter, you will have realized that fair tests of treatments have to be planned carefully. The documents setting out these plans are known as research protocols. However, the best-laid plans may not work out quite as intended – the treatments actually received by patients sometimes differ from those they were allocated. For example, patients may not take treatments as intended; or one of the treatments may not be given because supplies or personnel become unavailable. If such discrepancies are discovered, the implications need to be considered and addressed carefully.

During the 1970s and 1980s, there were remarkable advances in the treatment of children with acute lymphoblastic leukaemia, the most common type of leukaemia in this age group. However, it was puzzling that American children were doing substantially better than British children who, on the face of it, were receiving exactly the same drug regimens.[7] During a visit to a children's cancer centre in California, an astute British statistician noticed that American children with leukaemia were being treated far more 'aggressively' with chemotherapy than children in the UK. The treatment had nasty side-effects (nausea, infection, anaemia, hair loss, and so on) and when these side-effects were particularly troublesome, British doctors and nurses, unlike their American counterparts, tended to reduce or pause the prescribed treatment. This 'gentler approach' appears to have reduced the effectiveness of the treatment, and was probably a reason for the differences in British and American treatment success.

Helping people to stick to allocated treatments

Differences between intended and actual treatments during treatment comparisons can happen in other ways that may complicate the interpretation of tests of treatments. Participants in research should not be denied medically necessary treatments. When a new treatment with hoped-for, but unproven, beneficial effects is being studied in a fair test, therefore, participating patients should be assured that they will all receive established effective treatments.

If people know who is getting what in a study, several possible biases arise. One is that patients and doctors may feel that people allocated to 'new' treatments have been lucky, and this may cause them unconsciously to exaggerate the benefits of these treatments. On the other hand, patients and doctors may feel that people allocated 'older' treatments are hard done by, and this disappointment may cause them to under-estimate any positive effects. Knowing which treatments have been allocated may also cause doctors to give the patients who have been allocated the older treatments some extra treatment or care, to compensate, as it were, for the fact that they had not been allocated to receive the newer, but unproven treatments. Using such additional treatments in patients in one of the comparison groups but not in the other group complicates the evaluation of a new treatment, and risks making the comparison unfair and the results misleading. A way to reduce differences between intended and actual treatment comparisons is to try to make the newer and older treatments being compared look, taste and smell the same.

This is what is done when a treatment with hoped-for beneficial effects is compared with a treatment with no active ingredients (a sham treatment, or placebo), which is designed to look, smell, taste and feel like the 'real' treatment. This is called 'blinding', or 'masking'. If this 'blinding' can be achieved (and there are many circumstances in which it cannot), patients in the two comparison groups will tend to differ in only one respect – whether they have been allocated to take the new treatment or the one with no active ingredients. Similarly, the health professionals caring for the patients will be less likely to be able to tell whether their patients have received the new treatment or not. If neither doctors nor patients know which treatment is being given, the trial is called 'double blind'. As a result, patients in the two comparison groups will be similarly motivated to stick to the treatments to which they have been allocated, and the clinicians looking after them will be more likely to treat all the patients in the same way.

Fair measurement of treatment outcome

Although one of the reasons for using sham treatments in treatment comparisons is to help patients and doctors to stick to the treatments allocated to them, a more widely recognized reason for such 'blinding' is to reduce biases when the outcomes of treatments are being assessed.

Blinding for this reason has an interesting history. In the 18th century, Louis XVI of France called for an investigation into Anton Mesmer's claims that 'animal magnetism' (sometimes called 'mesmerism') had beneficial effects. The king wanted to know whether the effects were due to any 'real force', or rather to 'illusions of the mind'. In a treatment test, blindfolded people were told either that they were or were not receiving animal magnetism when in fact, at times, the reverse was happening. People only reported feeling the effects of the 'treatment' when they had been told that they were receiving it.

For some outcomes of treatment – survival, for example –

biased outcome assessment is very unlikely since there is little room for doubt about whether or not someone has died. However, assessing most outcomes will entail some subjectivity, because outcomes should and often do involve patients' experiences of symptoms such as pain and anxiety. People may have individual reasons for preferring one of the treatments being compared. For example, they may be more alert to signs of possible benefit when they believe a treatment is good for them, and more ready to ascribe harmful effects to a treatment about which they are worried.

In these common circumstances, blinding is a desirable feature of fair tests. This means that the treatments being compared must appear to be the same. In a test of treatments for multiple sclerosis, for example, all the patients were examined both by a doctor who did not know whether the patients had received the new drugs or a treatment with no active ingredient (that is, the doctor was 'blinded'), and also by a doctor who knew the comparison group to which the patients had been allocated (that is, the doctor was 'unblinded'). Assessments done by the 'blinded' doctors suggested that the new treatment was not useful whereas assessments done by the 'unblinded' doctors suggested that the new treatment was beneficial.[8] This difference implies the new treatment was not effective and that knowing the treatment assignment led the 'unblinded' doctors to have 'seen what they believed' or hoped for. Overall, the greater the element of subjectivity in assessing treatment outcomes, the greater the desirability of blinding to make tests of treatments fair.

Sometimes it is even possible to blind patients as to whether or not they have received a real surgical operation. One such study was done in patients with osteoarthritis of the knee. There was no apparent advantage of a surgical approach that involved washing out the arthritic joints when this was compared with simply making an incision through the skin over the knee under anaesthesia, and 'pretending' that this had been followed by flushing out the joint space.[9]

Often it is simply impossible to blind patients and doctors to the identity of treatments being compared – for example, when comparing surgery and a drug treatment or when a drug has a characteristic side-effect. However, even for some outcomes for which bias might creep in – say, in assigning a cause of death, or judging an X-ray – this can be avoided by arranging for these outcomes to be assessed independently by people who do not know which treatments individual patients have received.

Generating and investigating hunches about unanticipated adverse effects of treatments

Generating hunches about unanticipated effects of treatments
Unanticipated effects of treatments, whether bad or good, are often first suspected by health professionals or patients.[10] Because the treatment tests needed to get marketing licences include only a few hundred or a few thousand people treated over a few months, only relatively short-term and frequent side-effects are likely to be picked up at this stage. Rare effects and those that take some time to develop will not be discovered until the treatments have been in more widespread use, over a longer time period, and in a wider range of patients than those who participated in the pre-licensing tests.

In an increasing number of countries – including the UK, the Netherlands, Sweden, Denmark, and the USA – there are facilities for clinicians and patients to report suspected adverse drug reactions, which can then be investigated formally.[11] Although none of these reporting schemes has been especially successful in identifying important adverse reactions to drugs, there are instances where they have been. For example, when the cholesterol-lowering drug rosuvastatin was launched in the UK in 2003, reports soon began to identify a serious, rare, unanticipated adverse effect on muscles called rhabdomyolysis. In this condition, muscles break down rapidly and the breakdown products can cause serious kidney damage. Further investigation helped to show that the patients most at risk of this complication were those taking high doses of the drug.

Investigating hunches about unanticipated effects of treatments
Hunches about adverse effects often turn out to be false alarms.[10] So how should hunches about unanticipated effects of treatments be investigated to find out whether the suspected effects are real? Tests to confirm or dismiss suspected unanticipated effects

THE YELLOW CARD SCHEME

The Yellow Card Scheme was launched in Britain in 1964 after the thalidomide tragedy highlighted the importance of following up problems that occur after a drug has been licensed. Reports are sent to the Medicines and Healthcare products Regulatory Agency (MHRA), which analyzes the results. Each year, the MHRA receives more than 20,000 reports of possible side-effects. Initially, only doctors could file the reports, but then nurses, pharmacists, coroners, dentists, radiographers and optometrists were encouraged to do so. Since 2005, patients and carers have been invited to report suspected adverse reactions. Reports can be filed online at www.yellowcard.gov.uk, by post, or by phone.

One patient summarised her experience this way: 'Being able to report side effects through the Yellow Card Scheme puts you in control. It means that you can report directly without having to wait for a busy healthcare professional to do it . . . It's about putting patients at the centre of care. It's a quantum leap for patient involvement, and marks the beginning of the way forward and a sea change in attitude.'

Bowser A. A patient's view of the Yellow Card Scheme. In: *Medicines & Medical Devices Regulation: what you need to know*. London: MHRA, 2008. Available at www.mhra.gov.uk

must observe the same principles as studies to identify hoped-for, anticipated effects of treatments. And that means avoiding biased comparisons, ensuring that 'like is compared with like', and studying adequate numbers of instances.

As with hoped-for effects of treatments, unanticipated dramatic effects are easier to spot and confirm than less dramatic treatment effects. If the suspected, unanticipated treatment outcome is normally very unusual but occurs quite often after a treatment has been used, it will generally strike both clinicians and patients that something is wrong. In the late 19th century, a Swiss surgeon, Theodor Kocher, learned through a general practitioner that one of the girls whose thyroid goitre Kocher had removed some years previously had become dull and lethargic. When he looked into this and other former goitre patients on whom he had operated, he discovered that complete removal of the enlarged thyroid gland had resulted in cretinism and myxoedema – rare, serious problems resulting from lack of the hormone produced by the gland, as we now know.[12] The unanticipated effects of thalidomide (see Chapter 1, p4-5) were suspected and confirmed because the association between use of the drug in pregnancy and the birth of babies born without limbs was dramatic. Such abnormalities were previously almost unheard of.

Less dramatic unanticipated effects of treatments sometimes come to light in randomized trials designed to assess the relative merits of alternative treatments. A randomized comparison of two antibiotics given to newborn infants to prevent infection revealed that one of the drugs interfered with the body's processing of bilirubin, a waste product from the liver. The build up of the waste product in the blood led to brain damage in babies who had received one of the antibiotics being compared.[13]

Sometimes further analyses of randomized trials done in the past can help to identify less dramatic adverse effects. After it had been shown that the drug diethylstilboestrol (DES) given to women during pregnancy had caused cancer in the daughters of some of them, there was speculation about other possible adverse effects. These were detected by contacting the sons and daughters of the women who had participated in controlled trials. These follow-up studies revealed genital abnormalities and infertility in men as well as in women. More recently, when rofecoxib (Vioxx), a new drug for arthritis, was suspected of causing heart attacks, more detailed examination of the results of the relevant randomized trials showed that the drug did indeed have this adverse effect (see Chapter 1, p5-7).[14]

Follow-up of patients who have participated in randomized trials is obviously a very desirable way of ensuring that like will be compared with like when hunches about unanticipated effects of treatment are being investigated. Unfortunately, unless advance provision has been made for it, this is seldom an option. Investigating hunches about possible adverse effects of treatments would present less of a challenge if contact details of people who have been participants in randomized trials were collected routinely. They could then be re-contacted and asked for further information about their health.

Investigation of suspected adverse effects of treatments is made easier if the suspected adverse effects concern a totally different health problem from the one for which the treatment has been prescribed.[15] For example, when Dr Spock recommended that babies should be put to sleep on their tummies, his prescription was for *all* babies, not those believed to be at above average risk of cot death (see Chapter 2, p13-14). The lack of any link between the prescribed advice ('put babies to sleep on their tummies') and the suspected consequence of the advice (cot death) helped to strengthen the conclusion that the observed association between the prescribed advice and cot death reflected cause and effect.

By contrast, investigating hunches that drugs prescribed for depression lead to an increase in the suicidal thoughts that sometimes accompany depression presents far more of a challenge. Unless there are randomized comparisons of the suspect drugs with other treatments for depression, it is difficult to assume that people who have and have not taken the drugs are sufficiently alike to provide a reliable comparison.[16]

KEY POINTS

- Fair tests of treatments are needed because we will otherwise sometimes conclude that treatments are useful when they are not, and vice versa

- Comparisons are fundamental to all fair tests of treatments

- When treatments are compared (or a treatment is compared with no treatment) the principle of comparing 'like with like' is essential

- Attempts must be made to limit bias in assessing treatment outcomes

7 Taking account of the play of chance

THE PLAY OF CHANCE AND THE LAW OF LARGE NUMBERS

Trustworthy evidence about the effects of treatments relies on preventing biases (and of dealing with those that have not been prevented). Unless these characteristics of fair tests have been achieved, no amount of manipulation of the results of research can solve the problems that will remain, and their dangerous – sometimes lethal – consequences (see Chapters 1 and 2). Even when the steps taken to reduce biases have been successful, however, one can still be misled by the play of chance.

Everyone realizes that if you toss a coin repeatedly it is not all that uncommon to see 'runs' of five or more heads or tails, one after the other. And everyone realizes that the more times you toss a coin, the more likely it is that you will end up with similar numbers of heads and tails.

When comparing two treatments, any differences in results may simply reflect this play of chance. Say 40% of patients die after Treatment A compared with 60% of similar patients who die after receiving Treatment B. Table 1 shows what you would expect if 10 patients received each of the two treatments. The difference in the number of deaths between the two treatments is expressed as a 'risk ratio'. The risk ratio in this example is 0.67.

Based on these small numbers, would it be reasonable to conclude that Treatment A was better than Treatment B? Probably not. Chance might be the reason that some people got better in

	Treatment A	Treatment B	Risk Ratio (A:B =)
Number who died	4	6	(4:6 =) 0.67
Out of (total)	10	10	

Table 1. Does this small study provide a reliable estimate of the difference between Treatment A and Treatment B?

one group rather than the other. If the comparison was repeated in other small groups of patients, the numbers who died in each group might be reversed (6 against 4), or come out the same (5 against 5), or in some other ratio – just by chance.

But what would you expect to see if exactly the same proportion of patients in each treatment group (40% and 60%) died after 100 patients had received each of the treatments (Table 2)? Although the measure of difference (the risk ratio) is exactly the same (0.67) as in the comparison shown in Table 1, 40 deaths compared with 60 deaths is a more impressive difference than 4 compared with 6, and less likely to reflect the play of chance.
So, the way to avoid being misled by the play of chance in treatment comparisons is to base conclusions on studying sufficiently large numbers of patients who die, deteriorate or improve, or stay the same. This is sometimes referred to as 'the law of large numbers'.

	Treatment A	Treatment B	Risk Ratio (A:B =)
Number who died	40	60	(40:60 =) 0.67
Out of (total)	100	100	

Table 2. Does this moderate-sized study provide a reliable estimate of the difference between Treatment A and Treatment B?

ASSESSING THE ROLE THAT CHANCE MAY HAVE PLAYED IN FAIR TESTS

The role of chance can lead us to make two types of mistakes when interpreting the results of fair treatment comparisons: we may either mistakenly conclude that there are real differences in treatment outcomes when there are not, or that there are no differences when there are. The larger the number of treatment outcomes of interest observed, the lower the likelihood that we will be misled in these ways.

Because treatment comparisons cannot include everyone who has had or will have the condition being treated, it will never be possible definitively to find the 'true differences' between treatments. Instead, studies have to produce best guesses of what the true differences are likely to be.

The reliability of estimated differences will often be indicated by 'Confidence Intervals' (CI). These give the range within which the true differences are likely to lie. Most people will already be familiar with the concept of confidence intervals, even if not by that name. For example, in the run-up to an election, an opinion poll may report that Party A is 10 percentage points ahead of Party B; but the report will then often note that the difference between the parties could be as little as 5 points or as large as 15 points. This 'confidence interval' indicates that the true difference between the parties is likely to lie somewhere between 5 and 15 percentage points. The larger the number of people polled, the less the uncertainty there will be about the results, and therefore

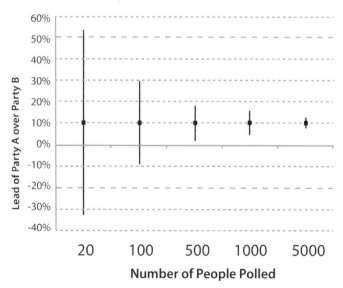

The 95% Confidence Interval (CI) for the difference between Party A and Party B narrows as the number of people polled increases.

the narrower will be the confidence interval associated with the estimate of the difference.

Just as one can assess the degree of uncertainty around an estimated difference in the proportions of voters supporting two political parties, so also one can assess the degree of uncertainty around an estimated difference in the proportions of patients improving or deteriorating after two treatments. And here again, the greater the number of the treatment outcomes observed – say, recovery after a heart attack – in a comparison of two treatments, the narrower will be the confidence intervals surrounding estimates of treatment differences. With confidence intervals, 'the narrower the better'.

A confidence interval is usually accompanied by an indication of how confident we can be that the true value lies within the range of estimates presented. A '95% confidence interval', for example, means that we can be 95% confident that the true value of whatever it is that is being estimated lies within the confidence interval's range. This means that there is a 5 in 100 (5%) chance that, actually, the 'true' value lies outside the range.

WHAT DOES A 'SIGNIFICANT DIFFERENCE' BETWEEN TREATMENTS MEAN?

Well, this is a trick question, because 'significant difference' can have several meanings. First, it can mean a difference that is actually important to the patient. However, when the authors of research reports state that there is a 'significant difference' they are often referring to 'statistical significance'. And 'statistically significant differences' are not necessarily 'significant' in the everyday sense of the word. A difference between treatments which is very unlikely to be due to chance – 'a statistically significant difference' – may have little or no practical importance.

Take the example of a systematic review of randomized trials comparing the experiences of tens of thousands of healthy men who took an aspirin a day with the experiences of tens of thousands of other healthy men who did not take aspirin. This review found a lower rate of heart attacks among the aspirin takers and the difference was 'statistically significant' – that is, it was unlikely to

WHAT DOES 'STATISTICALLY SIGNIFICANT' MEAN?

'To be honest, it's a tricky idea. It can tell us if the difference between a drug and a placebo or between the life expectancies of two groups of people, for example, could be just down to chance . . . It means that a difference as large as the one observed is unlikely to have occurred by chance alone.

Statisticians use standard levels of "unlikely". Commonly they use significant at the 5% level (sometimes written as p=0.05). In this case a difference is said to be 'significant' because it has a less than 1 in 20 probability of occurring if all that is going on is chance.'

Spiegelhalter D, quoted in: *Making Sense of Statistics*. 2010. www.senseaboutscience.org

be explained by the play of chance. But that doesn't mean that it is necessarily of practical importance. If a healthy man's chance of having a heart attack is already very low, taking a drug to make it even lower may be unjustified, particularly since aspirin has side-effects, some of which – bleeding, for example – are occasionally lethal.[1] On the basis of the evidence from the systematic review we can estimate that, if 1,000 men took an aspirin a day for ten years, five of them would avoid a heart attack during that time, but three of them would have a major haemorrhage.

OBTAINING LARGE ENOUGH NUMBERS IN FAIR TESTS OF TREATMENTS

Sometimes in tests of treatments it is possible to obtain large enough numbers from research done in one or two centres. However, to assess the impact of treatments on rare outcomes like death, it is usually necessary to invite patients in many centres, and often in many countries, to participate in research to obtain reliable evidence. For example, participation by 10,000 patients in 13 countries showed that steroid drugs given to people with serious brain injuries – a treatment which had been in use for over three decades – was lethal.[2] In another fair test organized by the same research team, participation by 20,000 patients in 40 countries showed that an inexpensive drug called tranexamic acid reduces death from bleeding after injury.[3] Because these studies had been designed to reduce biases as well as uncertainties resulting from the play of chance, they are exemplary fair tests, and provide good-quality evidence of great relevance to healthcare worldwide. Indeed, in a poll organized by the *BMJ*, the second of these randomized trials was voted the most important study of 2010.

The Figure below is based on data kindly provided by the award-winning team to illustrate how, to reduce the risks of being misled by the play of chance, it is important to base estimates of treatment effects on as much information as possible. The diamond at the bottom of the Figure represents the overall result of the trial of tranexamic acid. It shows that the drug reduces death from bleeding by nearly 30% (risk ratio just above 0.7). This

Death due to bleeding

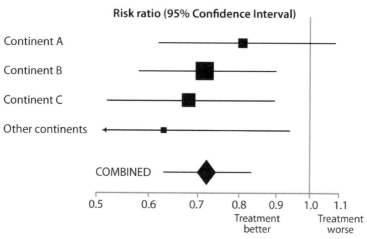

Effects of tranexamic acid on death among trauma patients with significant haemorrhage, overall and by continent of participants (unpublished data from CRASH-2: *Lancet* 2010;376:23-32).

overall result provides the most reliable estimate of the effect of this drug, even though the estimate from centres in Continent A suggests a less striking effect (which is not statistically significant, and likely to be an underestimate of the true effect) and the estimate from centres in the 'Other continents' category suggests a *more* striking effect (which is likely to be an overestimate).

In rather the same way that the play of chance can be reduced by combining data from many centres in a multinational trial, the results from similar but separate studies can sometimes be combined statistically – a process known as 'meta-analysis' (see also Chapter 8). Although methods for meta-analysis were developed by statisticians over many years, it was not until the 1970s that they began to be applied more extensively, initially by social scientists in the USA and then by medical researchers. By the end of the 20th century, meta-analysis had become widely accepted as an important element of fair tests of treatments.

For example, five studies in five different countries were organized and funded separately to address an unanswered, 60-year-old question: in premature babies 'What blood level of oxygen gives the greatest likelihood that babies will survive with no major disabilities?' If the blood oxygen levels are too high, babies may be blinded; if too low, they may die or develop cerebral palsy. Because, even in these frail babies, the differences resulting from different levels of oxygen are likely to be modest, large numbers are required to detect them. So the research teams responsible for each of the five studies agreed to combine the evidence from their respective studies to provide a more reliable estimate than any one of their studies could provide individually.[4]

KEY POINT

- Account must be taken of 'the play of chance' by assessing the confidence that can be placed in the quality and quantity of evidence available

8 Assessing all the relevant, reliable evidence

IS ONE STUDY EVER ENOUGH?

The simple answer is 'hardly ever'. Very seldom will one fair treatment comparison yield sufficiently reliable evidence on which to base a decision about treatment choices. However, this does sometimes happen. Such rare single studies include one showing that taking aspirin during a heart attack reduces the risk of premature death;[1] another making clear that giving steroids to people with acute traumatic brain injury is lethal (see below and Chapter 7, p89-90); and a third identifying caffeine as the only drug known to prevent cerebral palsy in children born prematurely (see Chapter 5, p57-58). Usually, however, a single study is but one of several comparisons addressing the same or similar questions. So evidence from individual studies should be assessed alongside evidence from other, similar studies.

One of the pioneers of fair tests of treatments, the British statistician Austin Bradford Hill, said in the 1960s that reports of research should answer four questions:

- Why did you start?
- What did you do?
- What did you find?
- And what does it mean anyway?

WHY DID YOU START?

'Few principles are more fundamental to the scientific and ethical validity of clinical research than that studies should address questions needing to be answered, and that they are designed in a way that will produce a meaningful answer. A prerequisite for either of these goals is that relevant prior research be properly identified. . . . An incomplete picture of pre-existing evidence violates the implicit ethical contract with research participants that the information they provide is necessary and will be useful to others.'

Robinson KA, Goodman SN. A systematic examination of the citation of prior research in reports of randomized, controlled trials. *Annals of Internal Medicine* 2011:154:50-55.

These key questions are equally relevant today, yet they are too often inadequately addressed or overlooked completely. The answer to the last question – what does it mean? – is especially important since this is likely to influence decisions about treatment and future research.

Take the example of a short, inexpensive course of steroid drugs given to women expected to give birth prematurely. The first fair test of this treatment, which was reported in 1972, showed a reduced likelihood of babies dying after their mothers had received a steroid. A decade later more trials had been done, but these were small and the individual results were confusing, because none of them had taken systematic account of previous, similar studies. Had they done so, it would have been apparent that very strong evidence was emerging favouring a beneficial effect of the drugs. In fact, because this was not done until 1989, most obstetricians, midwives, paediatricians and neonatal nurses had meanwhile not realized the treatment was so effective. As a result, tens of thousands of premature babies had suffered and died unnecessarily.[2]

To answer the question 'what does it mean?', the evidence from a particular fair treatment comparison must be interpreted

SYNTHESIZING INFORMATION FROM RESEARCH

More than a century ago, the president of the British Association for the Advancement of Science, Lord Rayleigh, commented on the need to set the results of new research in the context of other relevant evidence:

'If, as is sometimes supposed, science consisted in nothing but the laborious accumulation of facts, it would soon come to a standstill, crushed, as it were, under its own weight . . . Two processes are thus at work side by side, the reception of new material and the digestion and assimilation of the old; and as both are essential we may spare ourselves the discussion of their relative importance . . . The work which deserves, but I am afraid does not always receive, the most credit is that in which discovery and explanation go hand in hand, in which not only are new facts presented, but their relation to old ones is pointed out.'

Rayleigh, Lord. In: *Report of the fifty-fourth meeting of the British Association for the Advancement of Science; held at Montreal in August and September 1884*. London: John Murray, 1884: pp3-23.

alongside evidence from the other, similar fair comparisons. Reporting new test results without interpreting them in the light of other relevant evidence, reviewed systematically, can delay identification of both useful and harmful treatments, and lead to unnecessary research.

SYSTEMATIC REVIEWS OF ALL THE RELEVANT, RELIABLE EVIDENCE

Whilst it is easy to state that we should review the results of a particular study alongside other relevant, reliable evidence, this is a challenge in many ways. Reviews are important because people should be able to depend on them, and that means that they must be done systematically, otherwise they will be misleading.

THE IMPORTANCE OF SYSTEMATIC REVIEWS

'Systematic reviews and meta-analyses have become increasingly important in health care. Clinicians read them to keep up to date with their field, and they are often used as a starting point for developing clinical practice guidelines. Granting [funding] agencies may require a systematic review to ensure there is justification for further research, and some health care journals are moving in this direction. As with all research, the value of a systematic review depends on what was done, what was found, and the clarity of reporting. As with other publications, the reporting quality of systematic reviews varies, limiting readers' ability to assess the strengths and weaknesses of those reviews.'

Moher D, Liberati A, Tetzlaff, Altman DG. The PRISMA Group. Preferred reporting items for systematic reviews and meta-analyses: The PRISMA statement (www.equator-network.org), 2009.

Systematic reviews addressing what appears to be the same question about treatments may reach different conclusions. Sometimes this is because the questions addressed are subtly different, or because the methods used by the researchers differed; and sometimes it is because the researchers have introduced 'spin' in their conclusions. So, it is important to identify reviews that address the treatment questions that match those we are interested in; which are most likely to have been prepared in ways that reduce the effects of biases and the play of chance successfully; and which reach honest conclusions, in ways that reflect the evidence presented.

Reducing biases in systematic reviews

Just as biases can distort individual tests of treatments and lead to false conclusions, so they can also distort reviews of evidence. For example, researchers can simply 'cherry pick' those studies which they know will support the treatment claims they wish to make.

To avoid these problems, plans for systematic reviews, as for individual research studies, should be set out in research protocols. Protocols need to make clear what measures researchers will take to reduce biases and the effects of the play of chance during the process of preparing the reviews. These will include specifying which questions about treatments the review will address; the criteria that make studies eligible for inclusion in the review; the ways in which potentially eligible studies will be identified; and the steps that will be taken to minimize biases in selecting studies for inclusion in the review, and for analysing the data.

Identifying all the relevant evidence for systematic reviews

Identifying all the relevant evidence for systematic reviews – irrespective of the language or format of the relevant reports – always presents a substantial challenge, not least because some relevant evidence has not been reported in public. Under-reporting stems principally from researchers not writing up or submitting reports of their research for publication because they were disappointed with the results. And pharmaceutical companies suppress studies that do not favour their products. Journals, too, have tended to show bias when they reject submitted reports because they deem their results insufficiently 'exciting'.[3]

Biased under-reporting of research is unscientific and unethical, and there is now widespread acceptance that this is a serious problem. In particular, people trying to decide which treatments to use can be misled because studies that have yielded 'disappointing' or 'negative' results are less likely to be reported than others, whereas studies with exciting results are more likely than others to be 'over-reported'.

The extent of under-reporting is astonishing: at least half of all clinical trials are never fully reported. This under-reporting of research is biased and applies to large as well as small clinical trials. One of the measures that has been taken to tackle this problem has been to establish arrangements for registering trials at inception, and encouraging researchers to publish the protocols for their studies.[3]

Biased under-reporting of research can even be lethal. To their great credit, some British researchers decided to report in 1993 the results of a clinical trial that had been done thirteen

MARKETING-BASED MEDICINE

'Internal documents from the pharmaceutical industry suggest that the publicly available evidence base may not accurately represent the underlying data regarding its products. The industry and its associated medical communication firms state that publications in the medical literature primarily serve marketing interests. Suppression and spinning of negative data and ghostwriting [see Chapter 10, p124-5] have emerged as tools to help manage medical journal publications to best suit product sales, while disease mongering and market segmentation of physicians are also used to efficiently maximize profits. We propose that while evidence-based medicine is a noble ideal, marketing-based medicine is the current reality.'

Spielmans GI, Parry PI. *From Evidence-based Medicine to Marketing-based Medicine: Evidence from Internal Industry Documents. Journal of Bioethical Inquiry* 2010;7(1):13-29. Available online: http://tinyurl.com/Spielmans.

years earlier. It concerned a new drug for reducing heart rhythm abnormalities in patients experiencing heart attacks. Nine patients had died after taking the drug, whereas only one had died in the comparison group. 'When we carried out our study in 1980,' they wrote, 'we thought that the increased death rate in the drug group was an effect of chance... The development of the drug [lorcainide] was abandoned for commercial reasons, and this study was therefore never published; it is now a good example of "publication bias". The results described here...might have provided an early warning of trouble ahead.'[4] The 'trouble ahead' to which they were referring was that, at the peak of their use, drugs similar to the one they had tested were causing tens of thousands of premature deaths every year in the USA alone (see Chapter 2, p14-15).[5]

Reducing the play of chance in systematic reviews

In Chapter 7 (p91), we explained how the play of chance can be reduced by combining data from similar but separate studies – a process known as 'meta-analysis'. We used the example of five studies in five different countries organized and funded separately to address a 60-year-old quandary about what blood level of oxygen in prematurely born infants is needed to maximize the likelihood that they will survive with no major disabilities. That example illustrated how this process could be planned *before* the results of the studies were available, but the same process can be used *after* a group of similar studies have been completed.

For example, in 1974 a Swedish doctor conducted a systematic review of studies comparing the results of surgery for breast cancer with or without radiotherapy.[6] He found that, in all of the studies, women were more likely to die in the groups receiving radiotherapy. When all of this evidence was synthesized statistically using meta-analysis, it became clear that this excess mortality was unlikely to reflect the play of chance. Subsequent, more detailed analyses, based on evidence from individual patients, confirmed that the radiotherapy being used during that era did indeed increase mortality.[7] Recognizing this led to the development of safer practices.

Recognizing vested interests and spin in systematic reviews

What if the reviewers have other interests that might affect the conduct or interpretation of their review? Perhaps the reviewers have received money from the company that made the new treatment being tested. When assessing the evidence for an effect of evening primrose oil on eczema, reviewers who were associated with the manufacturer reached far more enthusiastic conclusions about the treatment than those with no such commercial interest (see Chapter 2, p18-20). However, commercial interests are not alone in leading to biased reviews. We all have prejudices that can do this – researchers, health professionals, and patients alike.

Disappointingly, people with vested interests sometimes exploit biases to make treatments look as if they are better than they really are (see also Chapter 10).[8] This happens when some researchers – usually but not always for commercial reasons –

deliberately ignore existing evidence. They design, analyze, and report research to paint their own results for a particular treatment in a favourable light. This is what happened in the 1990s when the manufacturer of the anti-depressant drug Seroxat (paroxetine) withheld important evidence suggesting that, in adolescents, the drug actually increased symptoms that prompted some of these young patients to contemplate suicide as a way of dealing with their depression.[9]

Over-reporting is a problem as well. In a phenomenon known as 'salami slicing', researchers take the results from a single trial (the salami) and slice the results into several reports without making clear that the individual reports are not independent studies. In this way, a single 'positive' trial can appear in several journals in different articles, thereby introducing a bias.[10] Here again, registering trials at inception with unique identifiers for every study will help to reduce the confusion that can result from this practice.

WHAT CAN HAPPEN IF ALL THE RELEVANT, RELIABLE EVIDENCE IS NOT ASSESSED?

Fair tests of treatments involve reviewing systematically all the relevant, reliable evidence, to see what is already known, whether from animal or other laboratory research, from the healthy volunteers on whom new treatments are sometimes tested, or from previous research involving patients. If this step is overlooked, or done badly, the consequences can be serious – patients in general, as well as participants in research, may suffer and sometimes die unnecessarily, and precious resources both for healthcare and for research will be squandered.

Avoidable harm to patients

Recommended treatments for heart attacks that had appeared in textbooks published over a period of 30 years were compared with evidence that could have been taken into account had the authors systematically reviewed the results of fair tests of treatment reported during that time.[11] This comparison showed that the textbook recommendations were often wrong because the authors

SCIENCE IS CUMULATIVE, BUT SCIENTISTS DON'T ACCUMULATE EVIDENCE SCIENTIFICALLY

'Academic researchers have been talking about something called "cumulative meta-analysis" for 25 years: essentially, you run a rolling meta-analysis on a given intervention, and each time a trial is completed, you plug the figures in to get your updated pooled result, to get a feel for where the results are headed, and most usefully, have a good chance of spotting a statistically significant answer as soon as it becomes apparent, without risking lives on further unnecessary research.'

Goldacre B. Bad Science: How pools of blood trials could save lives. *The Guardian*, 10 May 2008, p16.

had not reviewed the relevant evidence systematically. The impact of this was devastating. In some cases, patients with heart attacks were being deprived of life-saving therapies (for example, clot-busting drugs). In other cases, doctors continued to recommend treatments long after fair tests had shown they were lethal (for example, the use of drugs that reduce heart rhythm abnormalities in patients having heart attacks (see above and Chapter 2, p14-15).

The failure to combine the results of studies in systematic reviews as new evidence becomes available continues to harm patients. Blood substitutes that need no refrigeration or cross-matching are an obviously attractive alternative to real blood for the treatment of haemorrhage. Unfortunately these products increase the risk of heart attacks and death. Furthermore, a systematic review of the randomized trials reported since the late 1990s reveals that their dangers could and should have been recognized several years earlier than they were.[1]

Avoidable harm to people participating in research

Failure to assess all relevant, reliable evidence can also result in avoidable harm to people who participate in research. Researchers continue to be commissioned and allowed to do studies that involve withholding treatments known to be effective. For example, long after reliable evidence was available showing that giving antibiotics to patients having bowel surgery reduced their chances of dying from complications of the operation, researchers continued to do comparison studies that involved withholding antibiotics from half the patients participating in controlled trials. The researchers' failure to review systematically what was already known deprived half the participants in their studies of a known beneficial treatment. This serious lapse was evidently overlooked by the funding bodies who financed their research, and by the research ethics committees which reviewed the protocols and failed to challenge the researchers.

It is not only patients requiring treatment who can be put at risk if researchers do not assess systematically what is already known about the effects of the treatments they will be given. Healthy volunteers can be harmed too. The first phase of testing some treatments often involves a very small number of healthy volunteers. In 2006, six young men volunteers at a private research facility in West London were given infusions of a drug that had not previously been used in people. They all suffered life-threatening complications – one of them losing fingers and toes – and their long-term health has been compromised. This tragedy could most probably have been avoided[13] if a report of a severe reaction to a similar drug had been submitted for publication,[14] and if the researchers had assessed systematically what was already known about the effects of such drugs.[15] Had they done so, they might not have proceeded with their study at all, or if they had decided to go ahead, they might have injected the volunteers one at a time rather than simultaneously; and they could and should have warned the healthy young volunteers about the possible dangers.[16]

Wasted resources in healthcare and research

Failure to do systematic reviews of relevant, reliable research evidence does harm even when it is not harming patients and people participating in research. This is because it can result in resources being wasted in healthcare and health research. During

COULD CHECKING THE EVIDENCE FIRST HAVE PREVENTED A DEATH?

'In a tragic situation that could have been averted, Ellen Roche, a healthy, 24-year-old volunteer in an asthma study at Johns Hopkins University, died in June [2001] because a chemical she had been asked to inhale led to the progressive failure of her lungs and kidneys. In the aftermath of this loss, it would appear that the researcher who conducted the experiment and the ethics panel that approved it allegedly overlooked numerous clues about the dangers of the chemical, hexamethonium, given to Roche to inhale. Adding particular poignancy to the case is that evidence of the chemical's dangers could easily have been found in the published literature. *The Baltimore Sun* concluded that while the supervising physician, Dr. Alkis Togias, made "a good-faith effort" to research the drug's adverse effects, his search apparently focused on a limited number of resources, including PubMed, which is searchable only back to 1966. Previous articles published in the 1950s, however, with citations in subsequent publications, warned of lung damage associated with hexamethonium.'

Perkins E. Johns Hopkins Tragedy. *Information Today* 2001;18:51-4.

the 1980s and 1990s, for example, a total of more than 8,000 patients participated in several tests of a proposed new drug for stroke. Dutch researchers reviewed the results of these drug studies systematically, and were unable to find any beneficial effects (see Chapter 10, p121).[17] They then decided to review the results of tests of the drug done previously in animals; again, they were unable to find any beneficial effects.[18] Had the researchers who did the tests in animals and the clinical researchers reviewed the results of the animal studies systematically, as they had emerged, it is very likely that thousands of patients would not have been invited to participate in the clinical trials. Indeed, this might have resulted in better use of resources for treating patients experiencing stroke, and studies that were more likely to be relevant to identifying improvements in treatments for the condition. And this is far from an isolated example.[19]

REPORTS OF NEW RESEARCH SHOULD BEGIN AND END WITH SYSTEMATIC REVIEWS

The report of a study[20] to assess the effects of giving steroids to people with acute traumatic brain injury shows how to address all of Bradford Hill's four questions. The researchers explained that they had embarked on the study because their systematic review of all the existing evidence, as well as evidence of variations in clinical use of the treatment, showed that there was important uncertainty about the effects of this widely used treatment. They reported that they had registered and published the protocol for

---

INSTRUCTIONS TO AUTHORS TO PUT RESEARCH RESULTS IN CONTEXT BY THE EDITORS OF THE MEDICAL JOURNAL *THE LANCET*

Systematic Review

This section should include a description of how authors searched for all the evidence. Authors should also say how they assessed the quality of that evidence – ie, how they selected and how they combined the evidence.

Interpretation

Authors should state here what their study adds to the totality of evidence when their study is added to previous work.

'We ask that all research reports – randomised or not – submitted from Aug 1 . . . put the results into the context of the totality of evidence in the Discussion.'

Clark S, Horton R. Putting research in context – revisited.
Lancet 2010;376:10-11.

---

their study, when it started.

They described the measures they had taken to minimize biases and to achieve adequate control of the play of chance by studying a sufficiently large number of patients. They reported that their study had shown that steroids given to patients with serious brain injury increased the likelihood that these patients would die.

Finally and importantly, they provided readers of their report with all the evidence needed for action to prevent thousands of deaths from this widely used treatment because they updated their original systematic review of previous studies by incorporating the new evidence generated by their study.

KEY POINTS

- A single study rarely provides enough evidence to guide treatment choices in healthcare

- Assessments of the relative merits of alternative treatments should be based on systematic reviews of all the relevant, reliable evidence

- As in individual studies testing treatments, steps must be taken to reduce the misleading influences of biases and the play of chance

- Failure to take account of the findings of systematic reviews has resulted in avoidable harm to patients, and wasted resources in healthcare and research

9 Regulating tests of treatments: help or hindrance?

By now you will have realized that, all too often, careful evaluations of treatments do not happen and uncertainties about treatment effects persist unnecessarily. Perversely, as we commented in Chapter 5, some prevailing attitudes actively deter health professionals from working with patients to learn more about the effects of treatments. And, strange as it may seem, systems for regulating medical research in most countries contribute to this problem by forcing an artificial split between research and treatment. Research is assumed to be a highly risky activity requiring stringent oversight, whereas routine treatment

---

WHO SAYS MEDICAL RESEARCH IS BAD FOR YOUR HEALTH

'Most discussion about the ethics of medical research addresses the question of how research should be regulated. Indeed, medical research is in many ways much more strictly regulated than medical practice. From a perusal of the innumerable guidelines on medical research you could be forgiven for thinking that medical research, like smoking, must be bad for your health.'

Hope T. *Medical ethics: a very short introduction*.
Oxford: Oxford University Press, 2004, p99.

---

is regarded as much less problematic – even though, as we have described, patients can be put at risk by being given unevaluated or poorly evaluated treatments outside a research context.

Why is research seen as so risky and requiring special regulation, but routine treatment (which affects many more patients) is not? There is no ignoring a history of abuse by researchers, including experiments in which patients were exploited and used as a means to an end. And things do go wrong in research from time to time, so there is an available fund of horror stories. There is always the worry, too, that once people become research participants, their individual interests may become less important to health professionals than the overall interests of research.

The situation is further complicated by the highly variable motives of researchers: while some researchers conduct studies primarily to benefit the public, others are clearly motivated by money, or by enhanced career prospects. And sometimes it may be difficult to judge what the researchers' motives are. Research may therefore appear to be a scary prospect for patients and members of the public. It is partly because of this that there is a high level of regulation of research in healthcare.

Independent committees generally known as Research Ethics Committees (RECs, eg, in Europe) or Institutional Review Boards (IRBs, eg, in the USA) have helped to protect people from abuses perpetrated in the name of research. They review each research project and advise whether it can proceed or not, and play an important part in providing oversight of research and reassuring the public that approved studies have been designed with their interests at heart.

These committees are often made up of unpaid volunteers, including lay people. They review many different kinds of study protocols (the researchers' plans for what they intend to do) and also all the information that will be given to those who might take part in the study. The committees can require researchers to make changes to their protocols or to the information for participants. Without approval of the committees, studies will not go ahead. The committees therefore help to ensure that research participants are not put at unnecessary risk, and reassure participants and the public that researchers cannot simply do as they like.

Research is subject to many other forms of regulation. Laws specific to research exist in most countries. All countries in the European Union, for example, must comply with the Clinical Trials Directive, which lays out the requirements in relation to so-called 'clinical trials of medicinal products' – essentially this means drug trials. Several countries also operate regulatory systems that affect all or most types of research in healthcare. Many other laws can potentially affect research, even though they were not designed with research as their primary purpose. For example, data protection laws, intended to protect the confidentiality of people's personal data, apply, in many countries, to medical research. A range of different agencies is also usually involved in regulating research in most countries.

The conduct of research is also governed by professional codes of practice and by international statements. Doctors and nurses, for example, are bound by the codes of practice of their professional bodies, and can risk losing their registration or having other sanctions applied if they violate these codes. And international statements, such as the World Medical Association Declaration of Helsinki, are often highly influential in setting standards even when they have no legal force.

DO REGULATORY SYSTEMS FOR TESTING TREATMENTS GET IT RIGHT?

Although the level of regulation can be reassuring, current regulatory systems impose very onerous burdens on anyone wishing to study a poorly evaluated treatment rather than offer it to patients in normal clinical practice. In many countries, the sheer complexity of the system – involving laws, agencies, codes of practice, and so on – is overwhelming and time-consuming. Researchers may need to get multiple approvals from different places, and sometimes have to face resultant contradictory requirements.

Moreover, taken as a whole, the system can seriously discourage and delay the collection of information that would

IN AN IDEAL WORLD

'In an ideal world, wherever possible, we could be gathering anonymised outcome data and comparing this against medication history, making exceptions only for those who put their anxieties about privacy above the lives of others . . . In an ideal world, wherever a patient is given any treatment, and there is genuine uncertainty about which treatment is best, they would be simply and efficiently randomised to one treatment, and their progress monitored. In an ideal world, these notions would be so routinely embedded in our notion of what healthcare looks like that no patient would be bothered by it.'

Goldacre B. Pharmaco-epidemiology would be fascinating enough even if society didn't manage it really really badly. *The Guardian*, 17 July 2010. Available online: www.badscience.net/2010/07/pharmaco-epidemiology-would-be-fascinating-enough-even-if-society-didnt-manage-it-really-really-badly

make healthcare safer for everyone. For example, data protection laws and codes of practice on confidentiality, although introduced with the best of intentions, have made it extremely difficult for researchers to collect routine data from medical records that may help to pinpoint treatment side-effects. And for researchers planning clinical trials, it can take several years to get from a trial idea to recruiting the first patient, and even then recruitment to trials can be slowed by regulatory requirements. But while researchers try to get studies through the system, people suffer unnecessarily and lives are being lost.

In practice, what this means is that clinicians can give unproven treatments to patients, as long as patients consent, if therapies are given within the context of 'routine' clinical practice. By contrast, conducting any study of the same treatments to evaluate them properly would involve going through the protracted regulatory process. So clinicians are discouraged from assessing treatments fairly, and instead can continue to prescribe treatments without committing to

BIASED ETHICS

'If a clinician tries a new therapy with the idea of studying it carefully, evaluating outcomes, and publishing the results, he or she is doing research. The subjects [sic] of such research are thought to be in need of special protection. The protocol must be reviewed by an Institutional Review Board (IRB) [equivalent to a research ethics committee in Europe]. The informed consent form will be carefully scrutinised and the research may be forbidden. On the other hand, a clinician may try this new therapy without any intention of studying it, merely because he believes it will benefit his patients. In that situation, trying the new therapy is not research, the trial does not need IRB approval, and consent may be obtained in a manner governed only by the risk of malpractice litigation.

It would seem that the patients in the second situation (non research) are at much higher risk than are the patients in the first situation (being part of formal clinical research). Furthermore, the physician in the first situation seems more ethically admirable. The physician in the first situation is evaluating the therapy, whereas the physician in the second situation is using the therapy based on his or her imperfect hunches. Nevertheless, because ethical codes that seek to protect patients focus on the goal of creating generalizable knowledge, they regulate the responsible investigator but not the irresponsible adventurer.'

Lantos J. Ethical issues – how can we distinguish clinical research from innovative therapy? *American Journal of Pediatric Hematology/Oncology* 1994;16:72-75.

addressing any uncertainty about them (see Chapter 5).

The regulatory system for research, in its preoccupation with risk and protecting potential research participants, has become over-protective and overlooks the fact that patients and the public are increasingly involved as partners in the research process (see Chapter 11). However, there is one encouraging note. Research regulators are beginning to acknowledge that the 'one-size-fits-all' approach to research ethics review may be unnecessarily burdensome.[1] In the UK, for example, procedures for 'proportionate review' are now being evaluated to see whether a simplified and swifter review process can be safely used for research studies that do not raise any material ethical issues.

INFORMATION AND CONSENT

Requirements relating to provision of information and consent for studies are one of the ways in which the regulatory system acts to discourage rather than encourage research to address uncertainties about treatments. It is important – and ethical – to consider the interests of *everyone* currently receiving treatment, not just the few who participate in controlled trials.[2] The standard for informed consent to treatment should therefore be the same whether people are being offered treatment within or outside the context of formal treatment assessments. To come to a decision that accords with their values and preferences, patients should have as much information as they want, and at a time that they want it.

When treatment is being offered or prescribed in day-to-day practice, it is accepted that people may have different individual preferences and requirements, which may change over time. It is also recognized that people may vary not only in the amount or type of information they want, but also in their ability to understand all the information in the time available, and in their degree of anxiety

RETHINKING INFORMED CONSENT

'[Some] have come to suspect that informed consent is not fundamental to good biomedical practice, and . . . attempts to make it so are neither necessary nor achievable. We hope that the juggernaut of informed consent requirements that has been constructed across the last fifty years will be reformed and reduced within a far shorter period.'

Manson NC, O'Neill O. *Rethinking informed consent in bioethics.* Cambridge: Cambridge University Press, 2007, p200.

and fear. Health professionals are encouraged to help patients make choices about treatment in ways that are responsive and sensitive to what each individual wants at a particular time.

In research, however, provision of information to potential participants is overseen by regulatory agencies which often insist on the fullest possible disclosure of all potentially relevant information at the time that people are being invited to take part in studies. This may needlessly upset, frustrate, or frighten those who prefer to 'leave it to the doctor', or may raise needless concerns.[3]

The clinical trial of caffeine in premature babies that we mentioned in Chapter 5 (p57-58) provides a vivid illustration of how harm can be done by insisting that the fullest possible information be given to people who are candidates for research studies. The caffeine study recruited over 2,000 premature infants worldwide, but it took a year longer than expected because recruitment to the trial was slow. Recruitment was particularly

A COMMONSENSE APPROACH TO INFORMED CONSENT IN GOOD MEDICAL PRACTICE

'What is missing in the debate surrounding informed consent is the true nature of patient understanding, what information patients want to know, and how to deal with patients who wish to know only the minimum. There is little work in the area of assessing the understanding of the information given to patients. Clinicians often find it difficult to be certain how much patients or their relatives have correctly understood the information given to them. Understanding is affected by who is giving them the information, how it is explained, and the time or environment required to assimilate information. A paternalistic approach is unacceptable in medical practice; a common sense approach – explaining things clearly, tailoring what is said to what the patient seems to want, and checking understanding – is required for good medical practice.'

Gill R. How to seek consent and gain understanding. *BMJ* 2010;341:c4000.

slow in the UK, where several centres pulled out of the trial owing to regulatory delays in the approval process. On top of that, the research ethics committee insisted on parents being told that caffeine could cause fits in babies – when this complication had only been seen after a ten-fold overdose. So parents were being confronted by apparently frightening information that they probably did not need, and probably would not have been given if caffeine were to be used as part of routine treatment.

There is little evidence that widely promoted forms of research regulation do more good than harm.[4] Indeed, what evidence there is, is very disturbing. For example, in studies assessing the effects of treatments that have to be given without delay, requiring that the 'ritual' of written informed consent be observed can result in avoidable deaths as well as underestimates of the effects of treatments.[5]

Obtaining consent is a public health intervention which can do more harm than good. Like other well-intentioned interventions, its effects should be evaluated rigorously. The lethal consequences we have described might have been identified decades ago had the research ethics community accepted a responsibility to provide robust evidence showing that its 'prescriptions' are likely to do more good than harm.

A flexible approach to providing information for potential research participants, recognizing that trust between clinician and patient is the bedrock of any satisfactory consultation, is better than a rigid, standardized approach. But because of the way that regulatory systems intervene in research, clinicians are not currently free to choose how to explain research studies to patients. Moreover, they often find it difficult to talk about the uncertainties inherent in research. For example, as we mentioned in Chapter 5, clinicians recruiting patients to clinical trials often feel uncomfortable saying 'I don't know which treatment is best' and patients often do not want to hear it. Both doctors and patients therefore need a better appreciation of uncertainties and a better understanding of why research is needed (see Chapter 11).

ACADEMIC NICETY – OR SENSIBLE CHOICE?

'Twelve years ago I crossed the line between clinician and patient when, at the age of 33 years, I found out that I had breast cancer. At the time, I was doing a PhD about the problems of using randomised controlled trials (RCTs) to assess the effectiveness of treatments in my own discipline (orthodontics). During my research, I had become aware of the benefits of taking part in clinical trials and, ironically, the uncertainties about treating younger women with early breast cancer. So at the time of my diagnosis I asked my consultant if there were any RCTs that I could take part in. His response shocked me. He said that I "must not let academic niceties get in the way of the best treatment for me". But what was the best treatment? I certainly didn't know and also recognised that the profession was questioning what the optimum treatment was for early breast cancer in women younger than 50 years. So what was I to do?'

Harrison J. Testing times for clinical research. *Lancet* 2006;368:909-10.

WHAT REGULATORY SYSTEMS DO NOT DO

Although regulatory systems for research impose onerous requirements on researchers before studies start, there are many things they conspicuously fail to do, or do not do well. Many systems do not do enough to ensure that proposed studies are actually needed – for example, they do not require researchers to demonstrate that they have undertaken a thorough review of the existing evidence before embarking on new studies (see Chapter 8 for why systematic reviews are so important).

Moreover, most of the effort in regulating research is at the start-up stage, with the emphasis on controlling the entry of participants to studies. But there is surprisingly little effort devoted to monitoring studies once they are running, and to ensuring that researchers publish reports promptly at the end of their work (or even at all), stating how their findings have reduced uncertainty.

WHAT RESEARCH REGULATION SHOULD DO

'If ethicists and others want something to criticise in clinical trials, they should look at scientifically inadequate work, reinvention of wheels, and above all, unjustifiable exclusions and unjust and irrational uses of resources. The present debate is flawed by a failure to take note of what trials are for – to make sure that the treatments we use are safe, and do what they do better than the alternatives. There are no short cuts in ethics – no more than in trials.'

Ashcroft R. Giving medicine a fair trial. *BMJ* 2000;320:1686.

People who are invited to participate in research on the effects of treatments need to have confidence that the studies are worthwhile, and that their contributions will be useful. Regulatory systems need to do more to reassure them on both counts and dismantle needless barriers to good research directed towards research questions that matter to patients. There is a growing realization that testing treatments is everybody's business. As patients and the public take up the opportunities now being offered to become involved in planning and conducting research (see Chapter 11), they are likely to have an increasing voice in ensuring that regulatory obstacles are addressed.

KEY POINTS

- Regulation of research is unnecessarily complex
- Current systems of research regulation discourage fair tests of treatments that would make for better healthcare
- Despite the onerous regulatory requirements placed on researchers, regulatory systems do little to ensure that proposed studies are genuinely needed
- Research regulation does little to monitor and follow-up approved research

10 Research – good, bad and unnecessary

In earlier chapters we emphasized why tests of treatments must be designed properly and addressed questions that matter to patients and the public. When they are, everyone can take pride and satisfaction in the results, even when hoped-for benefits do not materialize, because important insights will have been gained and uncertainty lessened.

Although much health research is good – and it is steadily improving as it conforms with design and reporting standards[1] – bad and unnecessary research continues to be done, and published, for various reasons. And as for the perpetual demand 'more research is needed', a better strategy would be to do less, but to focus the research on the needs of patients, and so help to ensure that it is done for the right reasons. We explore these issues in this chapter.

GOOD RESEARCH

Stroke

Stroke is a leading cause of death and long-term disability. The death rate is between one in six and two in six during a first stroke, rising to four in six for subsequent strokes. One of the underlying causes of stroke is narrowing (stenosis) of the carotid artery, which provides blood to the brain. The fatty material that coats the inside of the carotid artery sometimes breaks away, blocking smaller arterial tributaries, and thus causing a stroke. In the 1950s surgeons began to use an operation known as carotid endarterectomy to remove these fatty deposits. The hope was that surgery would reduce the risk of stroke. As with any operation, however, there is a risk of complications from the surgical procedure itself.

Although carotid endarterectomy became increasingly popular, it was not until the 1980s that randomized trials were set up to assess the risks and benefits of surgery. Clearly this knowledge would be vitally important for patients and their doctors. Two well-designed trials – one in Europe and the other in North America – were carried out in patients who already had symptoms of carotid artery narrowing (minor stroke or fleeting, stroke-like symptoms) to compare surgery with the best available non-surgical treatment. Several thousand patients took part in these long-term studies. The results, published in the 1990s, showed that surgery can reduce the risk of stroke or death but that benefit depends on the degree of narrowing of the carotid artery. Patients with relatively minor narrowing were, on balance, harmed by surgery, which can itself cause stroke. These important findings had direct implications for clinical practice.[2, 3]

Pre-eclampsia in pregnant women

Another outstanding example of good research concerns pregnant women. Worldwide, about 600,000 women die each year of pregnancy-related complications. Most of these deaths occur in developing countries and many are linked to pregnancy-associated convulsions (fits), a condition known as eclampsia. Eclampsia is a devastating condition that can kill both mother and baby. Women with the predisposing condition – pre-eclampsia (also known as toxaemia) – have high blood pressure and protein in their urine.

In 1995, research showed that injections of magnesium sulphate, a simple and inexpensive drug, could prevent fits *recurring* in women with eclampsia. The same study also showed that magnesium sulphate was better than other anticonvulsant drugs, including a much more expensive one, in stopping convulsions. So, the researchers knew it was important to find out whether magnesium sulphate could prevent convulsions *occurring* in women with pre-eclampsia.

The Magpie trial, designed to answer this question, was a

MY EXPERIENCE OF MAGPIE

'I was really pleased to be part of such an important trial. I developed swelling at 32 weeks which grew progressively more severe until I was finally diagnosed with pre-eclampsia and admitted to hospital at 38 weeks. My baby was delivered by caesarean section and thankfully we both made a complete recovery. Pre-eclampsia is a frightening condition and I really hope the results of the trial will benefit women like me.' Clair Giles, Magpie participant.

MRC News Release. Magnesium sulphate halves risk of eclampsia and can save lives of pregnant women. London: MRC, 31 May 2002.

major achievement, involving more than 10,000 pregnant women with pre-eclampsia in 33 countries around the globe. In addition to normal medical care, half the women received an injection of magnesium sulphate and half a placebo (sham preparation). Magpie gave clear and convincing results. It showed that magnesium sulphate more than halved the chance of convulsions occurring. In addition, although the treatment did not apparently reduce the baby's risk of death, there was evidence that it could reduce the risk of the mother dying. And apart from minor side-effects, magnesium sulphate did not appear to harm the mother or the baby.[4, 5]

HIV infection in children

The results of good research are also making a real difference to children infected with HIV (human immunodeficiency virus), the cause of AIDS. At the end of 2009, figures from UNAIDS (the joint United Nations Programme on HIV/AIDS) show that an estimated 2.5 million children were living with HIV around the world, 2.3 million of them in sub-Saharan Africa. Every hour, around 30 children were dying as a result of AIDS.[6] Bacterial infections, such as pneumonia, which are associated with the children's weakened immune system, are a common cause of death. Co-trimoxazole is a widely available, low-cost antibiotic that has been used for many years to treat children and adults with chest infections unrelated to AIDS. Studies in adults with HIV additionally showed that the drug reduces other complications from bacterial infections.[7]

When preliminary evidence showed that the infections in children with HIV might also be reduced, a group of British researchers got together with colleagues in Zambia to assess the effects of co-trimoxazole as a possible preventive medicine in a large study. The trial, which started in 2001 and lasted about two years, compared the antibiotic with a placebo in over 500 children. The results became clear sooner than anticipated when it was shown that the drug cut AIDS-related deaths by 43% (74 deaths in the co-trimoxazole group compared with 112 in the placebo group) and also reduced the need for hospital admissions. At this point the independent committee scrutinizing the results recommended that the trial be stopped.

One immediate outcome was that all children in the trial were given co-trimoxazole as part of a Zambian government initiative. A wider consequence was that the World Health Organization and UNICEF promptly altered their advice on medicines for children with HIV.[8, 9]

These organizations continue to recommend co-trimoxazole as an inexpensive, life-saving and safe treatment for such children.[10]

BAD RESEARCH

Psychiatric disorders
Regrettably, research is not always well done or relevant. Take the example of a distressing condition known as tardive dyskinesia. This is a serious side-effect associated with long-term use of drugs called neuroleptics (antipsychotics), which are prescribed for psychiatric disorders, especially schizophrenia. The most prominent features of tardive dyskinesia are repetitive, involuntary movements of the mouth and face – grimacing, lip-smacking, frequent poking out of the tongue, and puckering or blowing out of the cheeks. Sometimes these are accompanied by twitching of the hands and feet. One in five patients taking a neuroleptic for more than three months experiences these side-effects.

In the 1990s a group of researchers began exploring, systematically, what treatments had been used for tardive dyskinesia over the preceding 30 years. Writing in 1996, they were rather surprised to have identified about 500 randomized trials involving 90 different drug treatments. Yet none of these trials had produced any useful data. Some of the trials had included too few patients to give any reliable results; in others the treatments had been given so briefly as to be meaningless.[11]

Members of the same research group went on to publish a comprehensive survey of the content and quality of randomized trials relevant to the treatment of schizophrenia in general. They looked at 2,000 trials and were disappointed in what they found. Over the years, drugs have certainly improved the prospects for people with schizophrenia in some respects. For example, most patients can now live at home or in the community. Yet, even in the 1990s (and still today), most drugs were tested on patients in hospital, so their relevance to outpatient treatment is uncertain. On top of that, the inconsistent way in which outcomes of treatment were assessed was astonishing. The researchers discovered that over 600 treatments – mainly drugs but also psychotherapy, for example – were tested in the trials, yet 640 different scales were used to rate the results and 369 of these were used only once. Comparing outcomes of different trials was therefore severely hampered and the results were virtually uninterpretable by doctors or patients. Among a catalogue of other problems, the researchers identified many studies that were too small or short term to give useful results. And new drug treatments were often compared with inappropriately large doses of a drug that was well known for its side-effects, even when better tolerated treatments were available – an obviously unfair test. The authors of this review concluded that half a century of studies of limited quality, duration, and clinical utility left much scope for well-planned, properly conducted, and competently reported trials.[12]

Epidural analgesia for women in labour

The importance of assessing outcomes that matter to patients is clearly illustrated – in a very negative fashion – by early trials of epidural analgesia given to women for pain relief during labour.

In the 1990s researchers reviewed the experience with controlled trials of epidural versus non-epidural analgesia. They estimated that, despite millions of women having been offered an epidural block over the preceding 20 years, fewer than 600 appeared to have participated in reasonably unbiased comparisons with other forms of pain relief. They identified nine comparison trials that could be confidently analyzed. The comparisons were commonly measured in terms of levels of hormones and other substances believed to reflect stress during labour. Outcomes for the baby were also the focus of some attention. Yet any comparison of the pain reported by the women themselves was absent in all but two of the trials. In other words, those conducting the trials had largely overlooked an outcome that was surely of supreme importance – how effectively a woman's pain had been relieved.[13]

UNNECESSARY RESEARCH

Respiratory distress in premature babies

Some research falls in between good and bad – it is plainly unnecessary. An example of such research concerns premature babies. When babies are born prematurely their lungs may be underdeveloped, with the risk of life-threatening complications such as respiratory distress syndrome. By the early 1980s there was overwhelming evidence that giving a steroid drug to pregnant women at risk of giving birth prematurely reduced the frequency of respiratory distress syndrome and death in newborn babies. Yet over the ensuing decade trials continued to be done in which steroids were compared with a placebo or no treatment. If the results of earlier trials had been reviewed systematically and combined using meta-analysis (see Chapters 7 and 8), it is unlikely that many of the later trials would have been started – the collective evidence would have shown that there was simply no need. These unnecessary studies therefore denied effective treatment to half the participants in these trials.

Stroke

Another example of unnecessary research, yet again because the results of preceding studies had not been gathered together and analyzed, concerns the treatment of stroke with a drug called nimodipine (one of a group of drugs called calcium antagonists). If it were possible to limit the amount of brain damage in patients who suffer a stroke, their chances of disability should be lessened. Beginning in the 1980s, nimodipine was tested for this purpose in stroke patients after some animal experiments had given encouraging results. Although a clinical trial in stroke patients published in 1988 suggested a beneficial effect, the results of several more clinical trials of nimodipine and other calcium antagonist drugs proved conflicting. When the accumulated evidence of clinical trials involving nearly 8,000 patients was reviewed, systematically, in 1999, no beneficial effect of the drugs was found (see Chapter 8, p102).[14] Since the use of nimodipine was apparently based on sound scientific evidence, how had this come about?

In the light of the results of research in patients, the findings from the animal experiments were scrutinized properly for the first time. Only when the animal studies were reviewed systematically did it become clear that the design of the animal experiments was generally poor and the results were beset by biases and therefore unreliable. In other words, there had been no convincing justification for carrying out trials in stroke patients in the first place.[15]

Aprotinin: effect on bleeding during and after surgery

Research funders, academic institutions, researchers, research ethics committees, and scientific journals are all complicit in unnecessary research (see Chapter 9). As we explained in Chapter 8, and as the first two examples of unnecessary research indicate, new research should not be designed or implemented without first assessing systematically what is known from existing research.

A shocking analysis published in 2005 focused on controlled trials of a drug called aprotinin to reduce bleeding during and after surgery. Aprotinin works. The shocking bit is that, long after strong evidence had accumulated showing that the drug substantially reduces the use of blood transfusion, controlled trials continued to be done.[16] At the time of the analysis, the reports of 64 trials had been published. Between 1987 and 2002, the proportion of relevant previous reports cited in successive reports of aprotinin trials fell from a high of 33% to only 10% among the most recent reports. Only 7 of 44 subsequent reports referenced the report of the largest trial (which was 28 times larger than the median trial size); and none of the reports referenced systematic reviews of these trials published in 1994 and 1997.

As the authors of the analysis emphasized, science is meant to be cumulative, but many scientists are not accumulating evidence scientifically. Not only are most new studies not designed in the light of systematic reviews of existing evidence but also new evidence is only very rarely reported in the context of updates of those reviews (see Chapter 8).

DISTORTED RESEARCH PRIORITIES

For most of the organizations supporting biomedical research and most of the researchers doing it, their stated aim is straightforward: to contribute information to improve people's health. But how many of the millions of biomedical research reports published every year really do make a useful contribution to this worthy cause?

Questions that are important for patients

Researchers in Bristol decided to pose a fundamental question: 'To what extent are questions of importance to patients with osteoarthritis of the knee and the clinicians looking after them reflected in the research on this condition?'[17] They began by convening four focus groups – of patients, rheumatologists, physiotherapists, and general practitioners, respectively. These groups were unanimous in making clear that they did not want any more trials sponsored by pharmaceutical companies comparing yet another non-steroidal anti-inflammatory drug (the group of drugs that includes, for example, ibuprofen) against a placebo. Instead of drug trials, patients wanted rigorous evaluation of physiotherapy and surgery, and assessment of the educational and coping strategies that might help patients to manage this chronic, disabling, and often painful condition more successfully.

Of course, these forms of treatment and management offer much less scope than drugs for commercial exploitation, and so are often ignored.

How many other fields of therapeutic research would, if evaluated in this way, reveal similar mismatches between the questions about treatment effects that matter to patients and clinicians, and those that researchers are addressing? Regrettably, mismatch appears to be the rule rather than the exception.[18, 19,20, 21]

Minor changes in drug formulation rarely lead to the drugs having substantially new, more useful effects, yet these types of studies dominate research into treatments not only for arthritis but also for other chronic disorders. What a waste of resources!

Who decides what gets studied?

Clearly this situation is unsatisfactory, so how has it come about? One reason is that what gets studied by researchers is distorted by external factors.[22] The pharmaceutical industry, for example, does research for its primary need – to fulfil its overriding responsibility to shareholders to make a profit. Its responsibility to patients and clinicians comes second. Businesses are driven by large markets – such as women wondering whether to use hormone replacement therapy, or people who are depressed, anxious, unhappy, or in pain. Yet only rarely in recent decades has this commercially targeted approach led to important new treatments, even for 'mass market' disorders. Rather, within groups of drugs, industry has usually produced many very similar compounds – so-called 'me-too' drugs. This is reminiscent of the days when the only bread available in supermarkets was endless variations on the white sliced loaf. Hardly surprising, then, that the pharmaceutical industry spends more on marketing than on research.

But how does industry persuade prescribers to use these new products rather than existing, less expensive alternatives? A common strategy is to commission numerous small research projects showing that the new drugs are better than giving nothing at all, while not doing any research to find out whether the new drugs are better than the existing ones. Regrettably, industry has little difficulty in finding doctors who are willing to enrol their patients in this fruitless enterprise. And the same doctors often

IMPACT OF 'ME-TOO' DRUGS IN CANADA

'In British Columbia most (80%) of the increase in drug expenditure between 1996 and 2003 was explained by the use of new, patented drug products that did not offer substantial improvements on less expensive alternatives available before 1990. The rising cost of using these me-too drugs at prices far exceeding those of time tested competitors deserves careful scrutiny. Approaches to drug pricing such as those used in New Zealand may enable savings that could be diverted towards other healthcare needs. For example, $350m (26% of total expenditure on prescription drugs) would have been saved in British Columbia if half of the me-too drugs consumed in 2003 were priced to compete with older alternatives. This saving could pay the fees of more than a thousand new doctors.

Given that the list of top 20 drugs in global sales includes newly patented versions of drugs in long established categories . . . me-too drugs probably dominate spending trends in most developed countries.'

Morgan SG, Bassett KL, Wright JM, et al. 'Breakthrough' drugs and growth in expenditure on prescription drugs in Canada. BMJ 2005;331:815-6.

end up prescribing the products studied in this way.[23] Moreover, drug licensing authorities often make the problem worse by insisting that new drugs should be compared with placebos, rather than with existing effective treatments.

Another strategy is ghostwriting. This is what happens when a professional writer writes text that is officially credited to someone else. Most people will have come across 'celebrity autobiographies' that have clearly been 'ghosted' in this way. However, ghostwritten material appears in academic publications too – and with potentially worrying consequences. Sometimes the pharmaceutical industry employs communication companies to prepare articles which, unsurprisingly, cast the industry's product in a favourable light. Once the article is ready, an academic is

DOCTORS AND DRUG COMPANIES

'No one knows the total amount provided by drug companies to physicians, but I estimate from the annual reports of the top nine US drug companies that it comes to tens of billions of dollars a year. By such means, the pharmaceutical industry has gained enormous control over how doctors evaluate and use its own products. Its extensive ties to physicians, particularly senior faculty at prestigious medical schools, affect the results of research, the way medicine is practiced, and even the definition of what constitutes a disease.'

Angell M. *Drug companies & doctors: a story of corruption.*
New York Review of Books, January 15, 2009.

signed up, for an 'honorarium', to 'author' it. Then the article is submitted for publication. Commentaries are especially popular for this purpose. Industry also targets journal supplements – separately bound publications that, while carrying the name of the parent journal, are often sponsored by industry and tend not to be as rigorously peer-reviewed as the parent journal.[24] Marketing messages created and promoted in ways such as these have led to the benefits of products being oversold and harms being downplayed (see also Chapter 8, p97).

Drug companies also place adverts in medical journals to promote their products. Typically these adverts include references to sources of evidence to back the claims being made. These may be convincing at first glance, but a different picture emerges when the evidence is scrutinized independently. Even when the evidence comes from randomized trials – which those reading the adverts might well assume to be a reliable assessment – all is not as it seems. When researchers analyzed adverts in leading medical journals to see whether the randomized trial evidence stacked up, they found that only 17% of the trials referenced were of good quality, supported the claim being made for the drug in question, and were not sponsored by the drug company itself. And it is known that research sponsored in this way is more likely

DODGY, DEVIOUS, AND DUPED?

Writing a light-hearted article for a Christmas edition of the *British Medical Journal*, two researchers created a spoof company called HARLOT plc to provide a series of services for trial sponsors. For example:

'We can guarantee positive results for the manufacturers of dodgy drugs and devices who are seeking to increase their market shares, for health professional guilds who want to increase the demand for their unnecessary diagnostic and therapeutic services, and for local and national health departments who are seeking to implement irrational and self serving health policies ... for dodgy "me too" drugs [our E-Zee-Me-Too Protocol team] can guarantee you a positive trial.'

To their astonishment, the authors received some apparently serious inquiries about the amazing HARLOT plc portfolio.

Sackett DL, Oxman AD. HARLOT plc: an amalgamation of the world's two oldest professions. *BMJ* 2003;327:1442-5.

to find a favourable outcome for the company's product.[25, 26]

Commentaries in prestigious medical journals such as *The Lancet*[27] have drawn attention to the perverse incentives now driving some of those involved in clinical research, and the increasingly dubious relationships between universities and industry. A former editor of the *New England Journal of Medicine* asked bluntly 'Is academic medicine for sale?'[28]

Commercial priorities are not the only perverse influences on patterns of biomedical research which ignore the interests of patients. Many people within universities and research funding organizations believe that improvements in health are most likely to stem from attempts to unravel basic mechanisms of disease. So, they do research in laboratories and with animals. Although such basic research is unquestionably needed, there is precious little evidence to support its substantially greater share of funding

ALL IT TAKES IS TO FIND THE GENE

'It's . . . hoped that the genetic revolution will cure every problem known to man. We will be able to locate and replicate the genes that predispose us towards building better housing, eliminating pollution, enduring cancer more bravely, implementing funds for universally available child-care facilities, and agreeing on the location and design of a national sports stadium. Soon, every newborn will be delivered on to a genetically level playing field. The gene that, say, makes girls do better at GCSEs [high school exams] than boys will be identified and removed. The genetic possibilities are endless. . . . So, yes we're entering an uncertain world, but one that holds out certain hope. For whatever the grave moral quandaries the genetic issue throws up, it will one day be possible to isolate the gene that solves them.'

Iannucci A. *The Audacity of Hype*. London: Little, Brown, 2009, pp270-1

than research involving patients.[29, 30] Yet the consequence has been a massive outpouring of laboratory research that has not been properly evaluated to see how relevant it is to patients.

One reason for this distortion is the hype surrounding the hoped-for clinical advances that basic research, especially genetics, might offer (see Chapter 4, p43-44 for genetic tests). Yet, as Sir David Weatherall, a distinguished clinician and genetics researcher, observed in 2011, 'Many of our major killers reflect the action of a large number of genes with small effects, combined with a major input from the physical and social environment. This work is producing valuable information about some disease processes, but it also emphasises the individuality and variability of the underlying mechanisms of diseases. Clearly, the era of personalised medicine based on our genetic makeup is a long way in the future.'[31]

Now, over fifty years after the structure of DNA was discovered, the cacophony of claims about early healthcare benefits of the 'genetic revolution' seems to be diminishing. Reality is starting to set in. One scientist, talking about the potential for genetics to

---

PSORIASIS PATIENTS POORLY SERVED BY RESEARCH

'Few trials involved comparison of different options or looked at long-term management. The duration of studies is unconvincingly brief in the context of a disease of potentially near life-long chronicity. We seem to know reliably only that our treatments are better than nothing at all. Tellingly, researchers have completely ignored patient experience, views, preferences, or satisfactions.'

R Jobling, Chairman, Psoriasis Association

Jobling R. Therapeutic research into psoriasis: patients' perspectives, priorities and interests. In: Rawlins M, Littlejohns P, eds. *Delivering quality in the NHS 2005*. Abingdon: Radcliffe Publishing Ltd, pp53-56.

---

result in development of new drugs, commented 'We have moved into an era of realism. . . . genetic aspects have to be looked at in association with other factors including environment and the clinical use of drugs. Just because a drug doesn't work in a patient doesn't indicate genetic variation in response is the cause.'[32] And an editorial in the science journal *Nature*, in an issue celebrating the tenth anniversary of the sequencing of the human genome, noted '. . . there has been some progress, in the form of drugs targeted against specific genetic defects identified in a few types of cancer, for example, and in some rare inherited disorders. But the complexity of post-genome biology has dashed early hopes that this trickle of therapies would become a flood.'[33]

There is simply no way of bypassing responsibly the need for well-designed research in patients to test the therapeutic theories derived from basic research. And, all too often, such theories are never followed through to see if they do have any relevance for patients. More than two decades after researchers identified the genetic defect leading to cystic fibrosis, people with the condition are still asking a fundamental question. When will they see dividends to their health resulting from the discovery?

Even when research may seem relevant to patients, researchers often appear to overlook patients' concerns when they design their studies. In a telling illustration, lung cancer doctors were asked to put themselves in the position of patients and to consider whether they would consent to participate in each of six lung cancer trials for which they might, as patients, be eligible. Between 36 and 89 per cent of them said that they would *not* participate.[34]

Similarly, in clinical trials in psoriasis – a chronic and disabling skin condition that affects about 125 million people worldwide – patients' interests have been poorly represented.[35, 36] For example, the Psoriasis Association in the UK found that researchers persisted in using a largely discredited scoring system in many studies to assess the effects of various treatments. Among its deficiencies, the scoring system concentrates on measures such as total area of skin affected and thickness of the lesions, whereas patients, not surprisingly, are more troubled by lesions on the face, palms and soles, and genitals.[37]

KEY POINTS

- Unnecessary research is a waste of time, effort, money, and other resources; it is also unethical and potentially harmful to patients

- New research should only proceed if an up-to-date review of earlier research shows that it is necessary, and after it has been registered

- Evidence from new research should be used to update the previous review of all the relevant evidence

- Much research is of poor quality and done for questionable reasons

- There are perverse influences on the research agenda, from both industry and academia

- Questions that matter to patients are often not addressed

11 Getting the right research done is everybody's business

In the preceding chapters we have shown how much time, money, and effort can be wasted in doing bad or unnecessary research into the effects of treatments – research that does not, and never will, answer questions that matter to patients. We hope we have convinced you that better testing of treatments in the future should come from productive partnerships between patients, clinicians, the public, and researchers.

HOW CAN PATIENTS AND THE PUBLIC HELP TO IMPROVE RESEARCH?

The formerly closed world of medicine is increasingly opening its doors to admit fresh ideas and former 'outsiders', and paternalism is steadily diminishing. As a result, patients and the public are contributing more and more to the conduct of healthcare research – both what is researched and how studies are undertaken.[1] Worldwide, there is growing support for collaborating with patients as partners in the research process, and useful guidance is now available for professionals who wish to involve patients and the public.[2,3,4]

Patients have experience that can enhance deliberations and provide insights. Their first-hand knowledge can shed valuable light on the way in which people react to illness and how this affects choice of treatments. Accumulating evidence from questionnaire surveys;[5] systematic reviews of research reports;[1]

PATIENTS' CHOICE: DAVID AND GOLIATH

'Who has the power to see that research questions actually address the greatest needs of patients in all their misery and diversity? Why aren't the most relevant questions being asked? Who is currently setting the questions? Who should be? Who shall direct this prioritisation? Patients are best able to identify the health topics most relevant to them and to inform their comfort, care, and quality of life, as well as its quantity. The patients are the David, who must load their slings against the Goliaths of the pharmaceutical companies who need evidence to market goods and make profits, and trialists who are driven by curiosity, the need to secure research money, professional acclaim, and career development. Profit, scientific inquiry, grant money, and research papers are acceptable only if the central motivation is the good of patients. Independent patients and organisations that advocate good quality research should ready their sling, carefully choose their stone, take aim, and conquer.'

Refractor. Patients' choice: David and Goliath. *Lancet* 2001;358:768.

reports of individual trials;[6] and impact assessments[7] shows that involvement of patients and the public can contribute to improving tests of treatments.

Among many initiatives, the Cochrane Collaboration (www. cochrane.org), an international network of people who review, systematically, the best available evidence about treatments, has embraced the input of patients from its inception in 1993. The James Lind Alliance (www.lindalliance.org), established in 2004, brings together patients, carers, and clinicians to identify and prioritize those unanswered questions about the effects of treatments that they agree are most important. This information about treatment uncertainties helps to ensure that those who fund healthcare research know what matters most to patients and clinicians.[8] Beginning in 2008, the European Commission

A KEY PARTNERSHIP

'People-focused research in the NHS simply cannot be delivered without the involvement of patients and the public.

No matter how complicated the research, or how brilliant the researcher, patients and the public always offer unique, invaluable insights. Their advice when designing, implementing and evaluating research invariably makes studies more effective, more credible and often more cost effective as well.'

Professor Dame Sally Davies. Foreword to Staley K. *Exploring impact: public involvement in NHS, public health and social care research.* Eastleigh: INVOLVE, 2009. Available from: www.invo.org.uk.

funded a project to promote the role of patient organizations in clinical trials with the aim of pooling experience among European countries through workshops, reports, and other exchanges.[9] In other countries, too, there is active public representation in research activities generally.

Roles are continually evolving[10] in various ways, enabling patients and the public to work together with health professionals, and new methods of doing so are being developed (see below *Bridging the gap between patients and researchers,* and Chapter 13, point 2, *Design and conduct research properly*).[11] This is happening across the whole spectrum of research activities:

- formulation of questions to be addressed
- design of projects, including selecting which outcomes are important
- project management
- development of patient information leaflets
- analysis and interpretation of results, and
- dissemination and implementation of findings to inform treatment choices.

INVOLVING PATIENTS IN RESEARCH

How has this involvement of patients in research come about? In Chapter 3 we showed, for example, how the treatment excesses formerly imposed on women with breast cancer led to challenges and changes, both from a new breed of clinician-researchers and then from patients. Clinicians and patients collaborated to secure the research evidence that met both rigorous scientific standards and the needs of women. When women challenged the practice of radical mastectomy they signalled that they were concerned about more than eradication of cancer: they demanded a say in the tactics employed to identify effective ways of dealing with the disease.

For those patients and members of the public who want to become fully involved as co-researchers, there are several possible avenues. For example, they can be involved individually or as a member of a health/disease support group, or they may participate in a facilitated group activity such as a focus group. Irrespective of the mechanism of their involvement, it will certainly help if they become familiar with the nuts and bolts of research methodologies so that they can contribute confidently and effectively in partnership with health professionals. And for this they will require good-quality information and training relevant to their role. We go on to explain in Chapter 12 why the way in which this information is presented, especially in terms of statistics, is critically important to proper understanding. There are also many less prominent ways in which patients and the public can contribute to research efforts, particularly if we can develop a culture of collaboration which accepts insights and observations from a patient's viewpoint.

Today's active patient-researchers can look back thankfully to the pioneering activity of early 'patient pioneers' who realized that they should speak up and challenge the status quo – and that to do so they needed accurate information. For example, in the USA in the early 1970s, a small group of breast cancer patients, led by Rose Kushner, set about educating themselves so that they could become effective. Then they started to educate others. Kushner was a breast cancer patient and freelance writer who, in the

LAY PEOPLE HELP TO RETHINK AIDS

'Credibility struggles in the AIDS arena have been multilateral: they have involved an unusually wide range of players. And the interventions of lay people in the proclamation and evaluation of scientific claims have helped shape what is believed to be known about AIDS – just as they have made problematic our understanding of who is a "layperson" and who is an "expert". At stake at every moment has been whether specific knowledge claims or spokespersons are credible. But at a deeper level, the stakes have involved the very mechanisms for the assessment of credibility: how are scientific claims adjudicated, and who gets to decide? [As this study shows,] debates *within* science are simultaneously debates *about* science and how it should be done – or who should be doing it.'

Epstein S. *Impure science: AIDS, activism and the politics of knowledge.* London: University of California Press, 1996.

early 1970s, challenged the traditional authoritarian physician-patient relationship and the need for radical surgery.[12] She wrote a book based on her thorough review of evidence of the effects of radical mastectomy. By the end of the decade, her influence and acceptability were such that she worked with the US National Cancer Institute reviewing proposals for new research.[13] Similarly, in the UK, lack of information prompted women to take action. For example, Betty Westgate set up the Mastectomy Association in the 1970s, and in the 1980s Vicky Clement-Jones founded the charity CancerBACUP (now part of Macmillan Cancer Support).

People with HIV/AIDS in the USA in the late 1980s were exceptionally knowledgeable about their disease. They were politically geared to defend their interests against the establishment, paving the way for patients to participate in the design of studies. This involvement ultimately led to a choice of treatment options being offered to patients in the studies and flexible designs to encourage participation. This example was followed in the early 1990s in the UK when an AIDS patient group was involved in studies at the Chelsea and Westminster Hospital, London: the patients helped to design studies.[14]

These AIDS activists made researchers sit up: what some researchers had viewed as havoc caused by organized patient groups was in fact a legitimate challenge to the researchers' interpretation of uncertainty. Until then, the researchers' approach had overlooked the patients' preferred outcomes. On the other hand, patients came to appreciate the dangers of making hasty judgements about the effects of new drugs and of demanding release of a 'promising' new AIDS drug before it had been evaluated rigorously. The researchers may have remonstrated that 'compassionate release' of new drugs in this way had merely prolonged the agony of uncertainty for current and future patients. However, the patients countered that it ultimately hastened the understanding of both patients and researchers about the need for unhurried, controlled evaluations of treatments, designed jointly, and taking account of the needs of both parties.[15]

In the 1990s, one AIDS trial provided a particularly clear illustration of the importance of patient involvement in research. This was at a time when the drug zidovudine had recently been introduced for the treatment of AIDS. In patients with advanced disease there was good evidence of a beneficial effect. The obvious next question was whether use of zidovudine earlier in the course of infection might delay disease progression and further improve survival. So, trials were begun in both the USA and Europe to test this possibility. The US trial was stopped early when a possible but still uncertain beneficial effect was found. With active participation and the agreement of patient representatives, and despite the US results, the European trial continued to a clear endpoint. The conclusions were very different: zidovudine used early in the course of infection did not appear to confer any benefit. The only clear effects of the drug in these circumstances were its unwanted side-effects.[16]

HOW PATIENTS CAN JEOPARDIZE
FAIR TESTS OF TREATMENTS

Involving patients in research is not always helpful in promoting fair tests of treatments. A survey of researchers in 2001 revealed some very positive experiences resulting from involving patients in clinical trials but it also laid bare some very real problems. These mostly resulted from everyone's lack of experience of this type of collaboration. First, there were often substantial delays in initiating research. There were also concerns about conflicting interests and 'representativeness' of some patients who had not yet appreciated the need to avoid bringing only their own interests to trial management meetings.[5]

Many of these problems seemed to arise from patients' understandable lack of knowledge about how research is done and funded. Desperate circumstances sometimes provoke desperate efforts to access treatments that have not been adequately evaluated and may do more harm than good, even to patients who are dying. We have already referred to the way that lobbying by patients and their advocates for 'compassionate' release of 'promising' new drug treatments for AIDS had its downside: it delayed the identification of treatments directed at outcomes that mattered to patients. More recently, counterproductive and misinformed advocacy, by both individuals and patient groups, has affected the prescribing of drugs for multiple sclerosis and breast cancer.

In the mid-1990s, interferons were introduced to treat patients with the relapsing-remitting form of multiple sclerosis on the basis of scant evidence of benefit. Very quickly, patients with all forms of multiple sclerosis clamoured for these costly drugs, and healthcare services agreed to fund their use. Interferons became an accepted standard treatment for this debilitating disease. As a result, we will never know how to give interferons appropriately in multiple sclerosis – the research was never done and it is now too late to turn the clock back. However, with the passage of time one thing has become abundantly clear – interferons have nasty side-effects, such as 'flu-like' symptoms.

Herceptin (trastuzumab), as we explained in Chapter 1, p9-12, is not a wonder drug for all women with breast cancer. Firstly,

PESTER POWER AND NEW DRUGS

'New drugs by their very nature are incomplete products, as full information about their safety, effectiveness and impact on costs are [sic] not yet available.

It is worth noting that enthusiastic support for what is "new" is not the sole preserve of newspapers and can often easily be seen in other media outlets and among the medical and scientific communities.

"Pester power" is a concept normally associated with advertising aimed at children. The question to be asked in this context is, are we witnessing patient pester power or quasi direct-to-consumer advertising, where awareness is raised about new products and patients, charities and indeed clinicians then demand that these products be made available? If this is the case, we need to know more about who is driving this type of marketing, its actual impact on clinician and consumer behaviours and whether it is permitted within the existing regulatory code of practice.'

Wilson PM, Booth AM, Eastwood A et al. Deconstructing media coverage of trastuzumab (Herceptin): an analysis of national newspaper coverage. *Journal of the Royal Society of Medicine* 2008:101:125-32

its effectiveness depends on a particular genetic make-up of the tumour, which is present in only 1 in 5 women with breast cancer. On top of that, the drug has potentially serious side-effects on the heart. Yet patient advocacy, fuelling a media frenzy, led politicians to go with the flow of public opinion: use of Herceptin was officially endorsed with scant regard for the existing evidence or acknowledgement that further evidence concerning the balance of benefits and harms was still awaited.

Patients' organizations: independent voices or not?

Another less well known conflict of interest exists in the relationship between patients' organizations and the

INVOLVING CITIZENS
TO IMPROVE HEALTHCARE

'The confluence of interest between advocacy groups, those who sell treatments, and those who prescribe them makes for a potent cocktail of influence, almost always pushing policy makers in one direction: more tests, more procedures, more beds, more pills. . .

As someone reporting in this field for more than a decade, I sense that what's often missing from the debate is a voice genuinely representing the public interest. Sponsored advocacy groups are quick to celebrate a new treatment or technology but slow to publicly criticise its limited effectiveness, excessive cost, or downright danger. And, like many journalists, politicians tend to be unnecessarily intimidated by senior health professionals and passionate advocates, who too often lend their credibility to marketing campaigns that widen disease definitions and promote the most expensive solutions.

The emergence of new citizens' lobbies within healthcare, well versed in the way scientific evidence can be used and misused, may produce a more informed debate about spending priorities. Such citizens' groups could routinely expose misleading marketing in the media and offer the public and policy makers realistic and sophisticated assessments of the risks, benefits, and costs of a much broader range of health strategies.'

Moynihan R. Power to the people. *BMJ* 2011;342:d2002.

pharmaceutical industry. Most patients' organizations have very little money, rely on volunteers, and get little independent funding. Grants from and joint projects with pharmaceutical companies can help them grow and be more influential, but can also distort and misrepresent patients' agendas, including their research agendas. The scale of this problem is difficult to gauge but a fascinating insight comes from a survey done to assess the level of corporate sponsorship of patient and consumer organizations working with the European Medicines Agency. This Agency coordinates the evaluation and monitoring of new drugs throughout Europe and, to its credit, has actively involved patient and consumer groups in its regulatory activities. However, when 23 such groups were surveyed between 2006 and 2008, 15 were shown to receive partial or significant funding from medicines manufacturers or pharmaceutical industry associations. Moreover, fewer than half of the groups accurately identified to the Agency the source or amount of funding that they received.[17]

In some cases patient organizations have been set up by drug companies to lobby on behalf of their products. For instance, one of the companies that makes interferon formed a new patient group 'Action for Access' in an attempt to get the UK National Health Service to provide interferons for multiple sclerosis (see above).[18,19] The message heard by patient groups from all of this publicity was that interferons were effective but too expensive, when the real issue was whether the drugs had any useful effects.

Bridging the gap between patients and researchers

We drew attention above to problems that can result from patients becoming involved in testing treatments, and ways in which they may unintentionally jeopardize fair tests. As with most things, good intentions do not guarantee that more good than harm will be done. Nevertheless, there are clear examples of the benefits of researchers and patients working together to improve the relevance and design of research. As a result, many researchers actively seek patients with whom they can collaborate.

In an example of the value of collaborative preparatory work, researchers explored with patients and potential patients some of the difficult issues involved in testing treatments given in an emergency. If therapies for acute stroke are to succeed, they need to be started as soon as possible after the stroke occurs. Because they were unsure of the best way to proceed, the researchers asked patients and carers to help them. They convened an exploratory meeting with a group of patients and health professionals, and conducted focus groups involving older people. As a result, plans for the trial were clarified and patients helped the researchers to draft and revise trial information leaflets.[20]

This thorough preliminary research led to plans for a randomized trial which were endorsed promptly by the research ethics committee. The focus group participants had recognized the ethical dilemmas of trying to obtain informed consent from someone with an acute illness which may well have left them confused, or unable to communicate, even if not unconscious. They were able to suggest solutions that led to an acceptable trial design for all parties, and substantial improvements in the information leaflets.

Social scientists are increasingly involved as members of research teams to formally explore sensitive aspects of illness with patients and so improve the way in which trials are done. For a clinical trial in men with localized prostate cancer, researchers wanted to compare three very different treatments – surgery, radiotherapy, or 'watchful waiting' – and this presented difficulties both for clinicians offering the trial and for patients trying to decide whether to participate in it. Clinicians so disliked describing the 'watchful waiting' option that they had been leaving it to last, and describing it less than confidently because they had mistakenly thought the men asked to join the trial might find it unacceptable. Social scientists were asked to study the issue of acceptability to help determine whether the trial was really feasible.

The social scientists' results were a revelation.[21] They showed that a trial offering 'watchful waiting' would be an acceptable third option if described as 'active monitoring', if not left until last to be explained by the doctor when inviting the patient, and if the doctors were careful to describe active monitoring in terms that men could understand.

The research, bridging the gap between doctors and patients, had identified the particular problems that were presenting difficulties for both parties and that could easily be remedied by better presentation of the treatment options. One result was that the rate of acceptance of men invited to join the trial increased over time, from four acceptances in ten to seven in ten. This more rapid recruitment meant that the effect of all these treatments for men with localized prostate cancer would become apparent earlier than would have been the case if the preparatory work had not been done. And, because prostate cancer is a common disease, many men stand to benefit in the future, earlier than they might have done.

WORKING COLLABORATIVELY BODES WELL FOR THE FUTURE

There are numerous ways in which patients and the public can become involved in testing treatments. As we have already outlined, they may be the prime movers – the ones who identify the gaps in understanding and the need to find new ways of doing things. Their input may be facilitated by researchers; they may be involved in some stages of the work but not others; they may be involved from the moment of identification of a specific uncertainty that needs addressing through to dissemination and implementation, and incorporation of the project's findings in an updated systematic review; and they may be involved in different ways within one project. Sometimes they initiate the work themselves. There is no hard and fast rule: the appropriateness of different strategies and approaches in a particular study will dictate those strategies chosen. As the localized prostate cancer trial described above illustrates, methods are evolving all the time – even within the course of a project.

When patients and researchers work together they offer a powerful combination for reducing treatment uncertainties for the benefit of all. Various methods for enabling this joint working, suited to individual studies as appropriate, with endorsement and support from national research organizations, bode well for the future.

KEY POINTS

- Patients and researchers working together can help to identify and reduce treatment uncertainties

- Input from patients can lead to better research

- Patients sometimes inadvertently jeopardize fair tests of treatments

- Relationships between patients' organizations and the pharmaceutical industry can result in distorted information about treatment effects

- To contribute effectively, patients need better general knowledge about research and readier access to impartial information

- There is no one 'right way' of achieving collaborative participation in research

- Patient participation should be appropriate for the specific research purpose

- Methods of involving patients are continually evolving

12 So what makes for better healthcare?

In the preceding chapters we have drawn together many examples to illustrate why treatments can – and should – be based on sound research designed to address questions that are important to patients. Whether we are members of the general public, patients, or healthcare professionals, the effects of treatments touch the lives of all of us one way or another. Robust evidence from fair testing of treatments really does matter.

In this chapter we look at how such evidence can shape the practice of healthcare so that decisions about the treatment of individuals can be reached jointly by clinicians and patients. Good decisions should be informed by good evidence, which will tell us about the likely consequences of different treatment options. However, the meaning and value of those consequences will be different for different individuals. So, using the same evidence, one individual may reach a different decision from another. For example, a fully functioning finger may mean a lot more to a professional musician, a good sense of smell to a chef, and good eyesight to a photographer than they would to other people. They may therefore be prepared to make greater efforts or take greater risks to achieve the result that matters to them. The interface between evidence and decisions is complex, so most of this chapter will address some common questions on this issue.

However, before that, we consider 'shared decision making' more closely and illustrate what it might look like in practice. Sharing decisions in this way steers a middle course between

SHARED DECISION-MAKING

'Shared decision-making has been defined as "the process of involving patients in clinical decisions". The ethos is one where professionals (should) work to define problems with sufficient clarity and openness so that patients can comprehend the uncertainties that surround most decisions in medicine and therefore appreciate that choices have to be made between competing options. The clinician's expertise lies in diagnosing and identifying treatment options according to clinical priorities; the patient's role is to identify and communicate their informed values and personal priorities, as shaped by their social circumstances.'

Adapted from Thornton H. Evidence-based healthcare. What roles for patients? In: Edwards A, Elwyn G, eds. *Shared decision-making in health care. Achieving evidence-based patient choice. Second edition.* Oxford: Oxford University Press, 2009, p39.

professional paternalism and abandoning patients to make up their own minds alone. Patients regularly complain about lack of information yet, quite naturally, they have different expectations of the responsibility they want to accept.[1, 2]

Some patients prefer not to have detailed information about their illness and treatment options and would rather leave things entirely to their professional advisers, but many are keen to learn more. For those who would like more information, there should be ready access to well-written material and to skilled health professionals who can advise how and where they can access it in a format that best suits them.

What constitutes an 'ideal consultation' can differ widely from one person to the next. Some people are content to adopt a dependent role while others prefer to lead. A more participatory role in coming to a decision – with the doctor's encouragement – can be the most rewarding approach and can become the preferred option once a patient experiences how this works. A simple question from a patient can open up the dialogue, as we illustrate below. Importantly, patients can be led to feel involved in their care when they are treated as equal partners, whatever the level of involvement.

WHAT MIGHT THE IDEAS IN THIS BOOK LOOK LIKE FOR YOU?

Although no two consultations are identical, the guiding principles for how to arrive at the best possible decision, as set out in this book, are the same. The goal is that both patient and health professional leave the consultation feeling satisfied that they have worked things through together in the light of the best available relevant evidence. Patients consult their doctors with a wide range of health problems – some short term; some long-term; some life-threatening; others just 'troublesome'. Their personal circumstances will be infinitely variable, but they will all have questions that need to be addressed so that they can decide what to do.

To illustrate this, we begin with a consultation between patient and doctor concerning a common problem: osteoarthritis ('wear and tear' arthritis) of the knees. We then go on to address some fundamental questions about using research evidence to inform

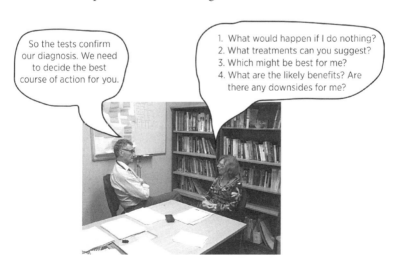

Dialogue between doctor and patient and some questions to ask.

practice – questions that patients with a wide variety of conditions might want answered when they consult a health professional, and those that readers of this book might well pose after reading earlier chapters.

SHARED DECISION-MAKING:
A CONSULTATION FOR A COMMON CONDITION

Doctor: Well, you have moderate osteoarthritis of the knees, which is common as people get older. It's often referred to as 'wear-and-tear-arthritis'. The usual course is for this condition to fluctuate – get better or worse – but with a slow progression over the years or decades. How is it currently troubling you?

Patient: Well, if I overdo things, my knees get quite painful and can stay that way for hours and make sleeping difficult. Recently, the pain has got worse, and I was worried I would need a knee replacement.

Doctor: Knee replacement is certainly an option but we usually reserve that for when simpler measures have failed.

Patient: So what else can you suggest?

Doctor: Well, simple analgesics or anti-inflammatory drugs can help manage the pain. Other than drugs, some special exercises to strengthen the muscles around the knee can help maintain function and decrease the pain. Would you like to know more about those?

Patient: Those drugs upset my stomach, so I'd like to hear more about the exercises.

Doctor: Fine. I'll give you a handout that explains some of the exercises, but also get you to see our physiotherapist. Meanwhile, you can safely take paracetamol regularly for the pain and stay active.

Patient: That's helpful, but aren't there more treatment options?

Doctor: There are further options available for severe osteoarthritis. But at this stage you could well find that you will experience a steady improvement as you build up the muscles with the exercises, sleep better because you have less pain, and can generally do more. You might also consider going swimming, or walking the dog more often, which will not only strengthen the muscles but should also help you 'feel good', and help to keep your weight in check into the bargain! I think we can safely leave considering more drastic options until we see how you get on with the exercises and the pain relief. But don't hesitate to come back to me if you think you're disappointed with progress.

QUESTIONS ABOUT TRANSLATING RESEARCH EVIDENCE INTO PRACTICE

Question 1: Isn't anything worth trying when a patient has a life-threatening condition?

It can be tempting to want to try the latest 'wonder-drug', or follow the example of some high-profile celebrity who has made claims in the popular press about a treatment regimen that they've followed, perhaps involving 'alternative' medicine that has been well-marketed but not tested. Mainstream treatments can seem much less glamorous and promising, but most that are being used for life-threatening conditions will have been painstakingly tested to find out how effective and how safe they are. So, seeking out the best evidence at the start can save much time, heartache, and money.

Mainstream medicine, generally speaking, recognizes that there are degrees of uncertainty about the effectiveness and safety of the medicines on offer. It aims to reduce those uncertainties to an acceptable level by testing, and by constantly and systematically reviewing the evidence to improve the treatments on offer. Such improvements depend critically on the help of patients who come to see that this is the only way to make solid progress.

Understandably, patients with life-threatening conditions can be desperate to try anything, including untested 'treatments'. But it is far better for them to consider enrolling in a suitable clinical trial in which a new treatment is being compared with the current best treatment. Such a comparison will not only reveal what extra benefits the new treatment might bring, but also what harms it might cause. Life-threatening conditions can need powerful treatments – and there is no treatment that does not have some side-effects. This makes it all the more important that a new treatment is tested thoroughly and fairly so that the findings can be recorded in a systematic way to see whether it is really likely to help patients.

Question 2: Although patients might want to know if a treatment 'works', suppose they don't want all the details?

It is important to strike a balance between information overload and depriving people of enough information to help them make an adequately informed choice. It is equally important to remember that a person may well need some information initially and more later on as they weigh the pros and cons needed to reach a decision. During a consultation, both doctor and patient should feel satisfied that the patient has the amount of information needed to go ahead and select, with the doctor, what the current best course of action is. But it doesn't stop there. If, after spending more time thinking about things, the patient has more questions and wants more details, the doctor should help the patient find out what they might want to know, and help clarify anything that is unclear.

Some choices involve difficult trade-offs; it may come down to choosing the lesser of two evils. For example, in Chapter 4 we discussed aortic aneurysm – the enlargement of the main artery from the heart – which may develop fatal leaks. Major surgery can correct the problem, but one or two patients per 100 will die from the operation itself. So there is a trade-off between the early mortality of the operation against the later risk of fatal rupture. Long term, an operation is the better bet, but some patients may reasonably choose not to opt for surgery, or at least delay it until after an important event such as their daughter's wedding. So rather than diving blind into an 'only hope' solution, it is better to weigh up the risks and their possible timing.

Question 3: Statistics are confusing – should patients really have to look at the numbers?

The way that numbers are presented can be very daunting – or even downright misleading. But if you really do want to compare one treatment with another, or to find out more about how the condition you have affects others like you, numbers always come into it somewhere. But some ways of presenting numbers are more helpful than others.

The best way to make the numbers mean something for lay people (and doctors too!) is to use frequencies. That means using whole numbers. So, saying 15 people out of a hundred is generally preferable to saying 15%. Then it is often helpful to give the numbers not only in words but also in graphic form of some kind – for example, coloured bar charts; pie charts; pin men/ smiley and sad faces in boxes, etc; and also in tables. Presenting 'numbers' with these 'decision aids' means that as many people as possible can grasp what the data mean.

Here is one way of explaining the effect of blood pressure drugs on the risk of heart disease and stroke in patients with high blood pressure over a period of ten years, using a bar chart.[3]

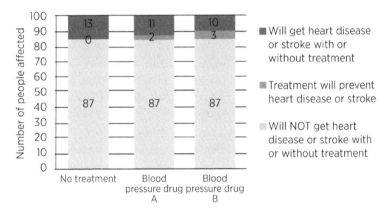

What will happen to 100 people like you in the next 10 years?

Out of 100 people with high blood pressure not taking any treatment, in the next ten years, 13 would be expected to get heart disease or have a stroke. If all 100 people took blood pressure drug A, only 11 of them would get heart disease or have a stroke – and two of them would avoid getting heart disease or having a stroke. If all 100 had taken blood pressure drug B, then ten would get heart disease or have a stroke and three would avoid getting heart disease or having a stroke. That's straightforward. Yet these simple numbers are often reported in terms only intelligible to statisticians.

Now let's look at how the numbers work out using a table rather than a bar chart. In this example we will concentrate on the better treatment – drug B:

Let's put the numbers into natural frequencies (simple counts) first, then work it through.

	NO TREATMENT	WITH DRUG B
Heart disease or stroke (over 10 years)	13 out of 100 people	10 out of 100 people
No heart disease or stroke	87 out of 100 people	90 out of 100 people
TOTAL	**100**	**100**

With no treatment, the risk of heart disease or stroke is 13% (or 13 out of 100), whereas with drug B the risk is 10% (or 10 out of 100) – a difference of 3% (or 3 out of 100). Since drug B prevents 3 of the 13 instances of heart disease or stroke that would have occurred, that is a relative risk reduction of 3/13 or about 23%. So we can say there was a 3% **absolute** risk reduction with treatment, or a 23% **relative** risk reduction. These are two different ways of expressing the same thing.

The relative risk reduction is always a high number – and sometimes a lot higher – and therefore is more attention grabbing. So if you see a headline saying '23% of strokes avoided' it tells you nothing – because it does not state the specific group of people affected, the timespan, or, most importantly, the risk of stroke without any treatment. It is most likely to be the relative risk reduction (but you need to check).

The numbers are sometimes very different. Consider the way a newspaper reported a study of prostate cancer screening. 'Could cut deaths by 20%' sounds large. The results could also have been expressed as one death prevented per 1,410 people screened (or a minuscule 0.07%, that is, seven premature deaths prevented per ten thousand men screened). The 20% is the relative risk reduction, the 0.07% the absolute risk reduction. The latter is much smaller,

---

**DON'T BE FOOLED
BY EYE-CATCHING STATISTICS**

'Let's say the risk of having a heart attack in your fifties is 50 per cent higher if you have a high cholesterol. That sounds pretty bad. Let's say the extra risk of having a heart attack if you have a high cholesterol is only 2 per cent. That sounds OK to me. But they're the same (hypothetical figures). Let's try this. Out of a hundred men in their fifties with normal cholesterol, four will be expected to have a heart attack; whereas out of a hundred men with high cholesterol, six will be expected to have a heart attack. That's two extra heart attacks per hundred.'

Goldacre B. *Bad Science*. London: Fourth Estate 2008, pp239-40.

---

because of the low rate of death from prostate cancer – and unlikely to have grabbed the headlines. The bottom line is that if a headline claim sounds overly optimistic it probably is![4]

So numbers do matter, and presented well can help people make decisions. Patients should not hesitate to ask their doctor to explain results in a way that they can readily understand – with visual materials for clarity as necessary. If decisions about treatments are to be shared, both doctors and patients need to be clear about what the numbers actually mean.

Question 4: How can someone know that the research evidence applies to them?

All decisions rely on previous experience of some kind – individual or collective. Fair tests of treatments such as randomized trials are simply well organized versions of that experience designed to minimize biases. Well organized or not, there will always be some uncertainty about how well previous experience can shape our advice for the next person. So if the patients who had been studied in the fair tests had a similar condition, at a similar stage or severity, to the individual in question, the most reasonable assumption is that the individual would get a similar response, unless there was a good reason to think they or their condition were substantially different.

Of course, even if the evidence is applicable, a patient might reasonably ask: 'people are all different so surely they may respond differently?' The 'fair test' of a treatment will only tell us what works on average, but rarely guarantees it will work equally well in everyone; and it cannot usually predict who will suffer unwanted side-effects. Research evidence can be used to guide what treatment is likely to be best, and then tried in an individual. With some skin rashes, for example, evidence-based treatment could be applied to one area of the body, using another area as a control (see Chapter 6, p74). By comparing responses in the two areas, both doctor and patient can tell whether it works, or whether there is an adverse effect. Indeed it's common to try a 'test patch' when first using some skin treatments, such as acne treatments on the face.

Mostly, however, we don't have the convenience of such a straightforward comparison. For some chronic and non-life-threatening problems, such as pain or itch, it is possible to try repeated periods on and off a drug in the same patient. This approach is also called an n-of-1 trial, meaning that the number (n) of participants in the trial is one – a single patient. With such tests in individual patients, the principles for a fair comparison that we outlined in Chapter 6 still apply, including an unbiased or blinded assessment of outcome, etc. Ideally, then, we would use placebo controls of skin treatments or pills, but this is often difficult to organize.

For many conditions, however, we cannot 'try it and see': the outcome is too remote or too uncertain. For example, it is impossible to know whether aspirin will prevent a patient's stroke until it is too late. This is a problem in most cases of preventive medicine, and also with treatments for many acute conditions, such as meningitis, pneumonia or snake bite, where we don't have the opportunity to test it in each individual patient and see. So we then have to rely on whether and how to apply the evidence from the experience of studying others.

In practice, if we are happy the evidence applies, it is then important to ask how the severity of the condition in the patient (or the predicted level of risk in those who are still well) compares with that of the people in the studies. In general, patients with more severe illness have more to gain from treatment. So if severity is equal to or greater than those in studies that showed a treatment to be beneficial, we can generally be confident about the applicability of the evidence. If their illness is less severe (or if still well, they are at relatively low predicted risk) the key issue is whether a smaller benefit than that seen in the studies might still be considered worthwhile.

Question 5: Won't genetic testing – and 'personalized medicine' – mean doctors can work out the specific treatment needed in every individual and make all this unnecessary?

Although the idea of being able to work out the specific treatment needed in every individual is undoubtedly attractive, and may be possible for a few conditions, it seems very unlikely that this approach will become the main way of treating people. As we explained when discussing genetic tests in Chapter 4 (p43-44) most diseases depend not only on complex interactions involving several genes, but also on the even more complex interactions between genes and environmental factors.

The results of genetic analyses have been important in informing decisions in families and individuals with inherited disorders, such as Huntington's disease, thalassaemias (inherited blood disorders), and some other (mostly rare) diseases. This genetic information has been a great boon in counselling families with these conditions. However, as far as the more common diseases to which we are all subject are concerned, genetic analysis adds little to information already available from family history and clinical examination. Although this situation is likely to change, our limited current knowledge means that we need to be careful not to overinterpret risks for common diseases predicted on the basis of genetic analysis.

We should declare that none of the authors have had their genetic profiles done, nor are we considering doing so. So it shouldn't surprise you that we would generally advise against genetic testing unless someone has (i) a family history that suggests a specific known genetic disorder, or (ii) one of the few currently known conditions in which a gene or genes clearly predicts who will respond to a treatment.

Question 6: If someone has a condition that is being studied in an ongoing clinical trial, how do they find out about this if their doctor doesn't know about it? (See also Additional Resources)

Fewer than one in 100 people seeing a doctor will be enrolled in a clinical trial. The proportion varies widely by condition and setting. Even within cancer centres – where trials are widely accepted and used – the range is enormous: most children with cancer are enrolled in trials, but fewer than one in ten adults are. Most trial enrolment depends on the centre a patient is attending: if the centre is not involved in the trial then they won't be able to enrol patients. So patients might need to look for a centre that is involved in clinical trials. There are a few community-based trials where patients can enrol directly; for example, these often occur in research designed to find out how to help people with mental health problems, such as depression or anxiety. More recently, some other trials have enrolled people directly through the internet. For example, a recent study to assess the effects of stretching before exercise enrolled all participants in this way: they never attended a clinic, but received all their instructions and follow-up over the internet.

If their doctors seem reluctant to enrol patients in trials, patients should find out why. It may be that the patient is not really eligible, for example. However, it may be simply that the doctor is put off by the extra work imposed by the burdensome regulatory demands (see Chapter 9). Patients who believe that they are likely to be eligible for participation in ongoing trials should persist. If a suitable trial is known to exist and a patient makes it clear that they are keen to be enrolled, doctors should support this.

Question 7: What's the best way of telling if the evidence (on the web or elsewhere) is reliable? What should people look out for?

Unfortunately there is no completely reliable simple marker for reliable information. If you are not going to look at the original research yourself, you are putting your trust in someone else's assessment. So it is important to assess the likely competence of that person (or organization) and to note whether there is a conflict of interest (or an axe to grind). If not, then ask yourself whether you trust them to have found and assessed the best research: is it described and referenced?

For example, suppose someone wanted to know whether beta-carotene (related to Vitamin A) increases or decreases the risk of cancer. A Google search for 'beta-carotene cancer' brings over 800,000 results. Looking at the first ten there are four primary research studies and six that are reviews or opinions. Of those six, there are three that have advertisements for vitamins or alternative medicines on the same page: a worrying sign.

One of these poorer websites says:

'Question: Does beta-carotene prevent cancer? Answer: Studies have shown that beta-carotene can help reduce the risk of cancer. Beta-carotene can be found in yellow, red, and deep green vegetables. It is also found in fruits. It is a common belief that taking a beta-carotene supplement will have the same effect as eating fruits and vegetables that contain it. However, this is not the case. Studies found an increased lung cancer risk among study participants.'

In addition to the advertisements, 'studies' are mentioned but with no description of them or references to published studies – that is a warning sign. It is impossible to tell whether or not the writer has searched for and appraised the 'studies' or merely stumbled on ones where he or she liked the conclusions.

Contrast this with the Wikipedia entry (also in the first ten):

'A review of all randomized controlled trials in the scientific literature by the Cochrane Collaboration published in JAMA in 2007 found that β-carotene increased mortality by something between 1 and 8% (Relative Risk 1.05, 95% confidence interval 1.01-1.08).[15] However, this meta-analysis included two large studies of smokers, so it is not clear that the results apply to the general population.[16]'

This entry states the type of evidence (randomized trials), and gives the references (the numbers in the square brackets). So, the fact that there are no advertisements, and there are specific details about the evidence, is reassuring.

Question 8: Are there reliable sources of information that can be recommended? (See also Additional Resources)

There is no single information source for all diseases and treatments. To apply the principles in this book, readers may want to develop some skills themselves. For example, in addition to Chapters 6-8 in this book, the book *Smart Health Choices*[5] gives some tips on how to find good information, and what to check for.

Of the websites available, few are largely based on systematic reviews. Some that are include the Cochrane Database of Systematic Reviews (www.cochrane.org/cochrane-reviews), which has lay summaries, and the IQWIG website (in German, but also translated into English at www.informedhealthonline.org). In addition, there are many websites that generally provide good information but are not always based on systematic reviews of the best available evidence – for example, NHS Choices (www.nhs.uk) and PubMed Health (www.pubmed.gov/health) both provide high-quality information.

Of course, there is also a lot to be wary of. In particular, watch out for conflicts of interest, such as sites that might financially benefit from people believing the information or others that try to sell something. This can be hard to detect, however – for example, as we mentioned in Chapter 11, some patient groups have undeclared funding from pharmaceutical companies and that can taint the information provided.

Question 9: How should people avoid being 'labelled' with an 'illness' and getting unnecessary treatments?

Medicine has made amazing advances: vaccines and antibiotics for preventing and treating infections; joint replacements; cataract surgery; and treatment of childhood cancers, to name but a few. But that success encourages medicine to extend its reach to areas of less benefit. To a person with a hammer, the whole world looks like a nail; and to a doctor (or a drug company!) with a new treatment everything looks like an illness. For example, as better treatments for diabetes and high blood pressure have become available, the temptation is for doctors to suggest their use to patients with only slightly abnormal results. This dramatically increases the number of people labelled as diabetic or hypertensive, 'medicalizing' many people who once would have been classed as normal.

In addition to any adverse effects of (sometimes unnecessary) treatment, this 'labelling' has both psychological and social consequences, which can affect a person's sense of well being, as well as creating problems with employment or insurance. So it is important for patients and the public to recognize this chain of events; to pause and consider the likely balance of harms and benefits before too hastily agreeing to a treatment. As we discussed in Chapter 4, screening commonly causes these problems of labelling through overdiagnosis, and potential overtreatment.

The first defence is to be wary of labels and proposed further investigations. The seemingly flippant remark that a normal person is someone who has not been investigated enough has a very serious side to it. So it is always wise to ask whether the

---

WHO HAS DIABETES?

So how do we decide who has diabetes? When I was in medical school, our numerical rule was this: if you had a fasting blood sugar over 140, then you had diabetes. But in 1997 the Expert Committee on the Diagnosis and Classification of Diabetes Mellitus redefined the disorder. Now if you have a fasting blood sugar over 126, you have diabetes. So everyone who has a blood sugar between 126 and 140 used to be normal but now has diabetes. That little change turned over 1.6 million people into patients.

Is that a problem? Maybe, maybe not. Because we changed the rules, we now treat more patients for diabetes. That may mean we have lowered the chance of diabetic complications for some of these new patients. But because these patients have milder diabetes (relatively low blood sugars between 126 and 140), they are at relatively low risk of these complications to begin with.

Welch HG, Schwartz LM, Woloshin S. *Overdiagnosed: making people sick in the pursuit of health.* Boston: Beacon Press, 2011: p17-18.

---

illness is considered high or low risk. And, as we suggested earlier, also to ask what would happen if nothing immediate was done: how might the condition be monitored, and what would be the signal for action? Some doctors are relieved that patients don't want immediate treatment or tests. But other doctors fall into the labelling trap – label = disease = mandatory treatment – not realizing that the patient may be quite happy to wait and see if the problem gets better or worse by itself.

WHERE DO WE GO FROM HERE?

The issues discussed above – about individual concerns and values, about understanding statistics and how they apply to individuals, and about the concerns of extending effective treatments to increasingly milder degrees of disease – all speak to a need for better communication between patient and doctor, and between the health sector and the citizens it serves. So we will finish this chapter with the Salzburg Statement on shared decision making, which sets out an agenda for different groups to improve how we work together.[6, 7]

Salzburg statement on shared decision making

We call on clinicians to:

- Recognize that they have an ethical imperative to share important decisions with patients
- Stimulate a two way flow of information and encourage patients to ask questions, explain their circumstances, and express their personal preferences
- Provide accurate information about options and the uncertainties, benefits, and harms of treatment in line with best practice for risk communication
- Tailor information to individual patient needs and allow them sufficient time to consider their options
- Acknowledge that most decisions do not have to be taken immediately, and give patients and their families the resources and help to reach decisions

---

We call on clinicians, researchers, editors, journalists, and others to:

- Ensure that the information they provide is clear, evidence based, and up to date and that conflicts of interest are declared

We call on patients to:

- Speak up about their concerns, questions, and what's important to them
- Recognize that they have a right to be equal participants in their care
- Seek and use high quality health information

We call on policy makers to:

- Adopt policies that encourage shared decision making, including its measurement, as a stimulus for improvement
- Amend informed consent laws to support the development of skills and tools for shared decision making

Why

- Much of the care patients receive is based on the ability and readiness of individual clinicians to provide it, rather than on widely agreed standards of best practice or patients' preferences for treatment
- Clinicians are often slow to recognize the extent to which patients wish to be involved in understanding their health problems, in knowing the options available to them, and in making decisions that take account of their personal preferences
- Many patients and their families find it difficult to take an active part in healthcare decisions. Some lack the confidence to question health professionals. Many have only a limited understanding about health and its determinants and do not know where to find information that is clear, trustworthy, and easy to understand

13 Research for the right reasons: blueprint for a better future

Medical research has undoubtedly contributed to better quality of life and increased longevity. Nevertheless, we have illustrated in this book how the existing 'drivers' for research – commercial and academic – have not done enough to identify and address patients' priorities.

Huge sums of money – over $100 billion every year worldwide – are spent on funding medical research.[1] However, most of this funding is invested in laboratory and animal studies, rather than in studies that are likely to produce evidence more immediately relevant to patients.

Even when it comes to deciding which questions about the effects of treatments will be studied, patients' priorities are widely ignored. The drug industry's financial power means it is very influential in decisions about what gets researched. Because industry can pay handsomely (thousands of pounds/dollars) for each patient recruited to its clinical trials, academics – and the institutions they work in – too often take part in clinical trials that address questions of interest to industry rather than to patients.

Regrettably, much of the money spent on medical research is wasted at successive stages – by asking the wrong research questions; by doing studies that are unnecessary or poorly designed; by failing to publish and make accessible the research results in full; and by producing biased and unhelpful research reports. This should matter to everyone – researchers, research funders, clinicians, tax payers, and above all patients.

Before setting out our blueprint for a better future, we briefly outline why, if research is to be better, it is vitally important to:

1. Ask the right research questions
2. Design and conduct research properly
3. Publish all the results and make them accessible
4. Produce unbiased and useful research reports

Waste at four stages of research

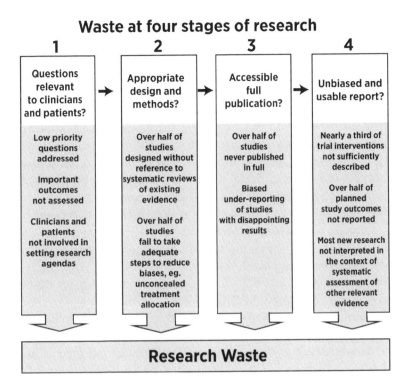

1	2	3	4
Questions relevant to clinicians and patients?	Appropriate design and methods?	Accessible full publication?	Unbiased and usable report?
Low priority questions addressed	Over half of studies designed without reference to systematic reviews of existing evidence	Over half of studies never published in full	Nearly a third of trial interventions not sufficiently described
Important outcomes not assessed		Biased under-reporting of studies with disappointing results	Over half of planned study outcomes not reported
Clinicians and patients not involved in setting research agendas	Over half of studies fail to take adequate steps to reduce biases, eg. unconcealed treatment allocation		Most new research not interpreted in the context of systematic assessment of other relevant evidence

Research Waste

How the money spent on medical research is wasted at successive stages.[1]

1. Ask the right research questions

Sometimes doctors do not know which treatment is likely to be best for their patients because the available options have not been properly studied. Such studies, which can have important implications for patient care, may be of little or no interest to industry or academia so important questions remain unanswered. And not answering these questions can lead to immense harm. Take one example – whether steroid drugs given to people with brain damage as a result of physical injury increase or decrease their chances of survival. Steroids were used for decades before a well-designed study showed that this established treatment had probably been killing thousands of patients with brain injury.[2] Proposals for this study were initially opposed by industry

161

and some university researchers. Why? They were engaged in commercial trials assessing the effects of expensive new drugs (so-called neuroprotective agents) on outcome measures of questionable importance to patients, and they did not wish to face competition for participants.

Another reason for tackling these unanswered questions is to help ensure that the precious resources available for healthcare are not being wasted. When human albumin solution, given as an intravenous drip, was introduced during the 1940s to resuscitate burned and other critically ill patients, theory suggested that it should reduce their chances of dying. Amazingly, this theory was not subjected to fair tests until the 1990s. At that point, a systematic review of the relevant randomized trials could find no evidence that human albumin solution reduced the risk of death compared with simple salt solutions. What the systematic review showed, in fact, was that if albumin had any effect on death risk it was to increase it.[3] The findings in this review prompted doctors in Australia and New Zealand to get together to do the first sufficiently large fair comparison of human albumin solution with saline (salt water), an alternative resuscitation fluid.[4] This study – which should have been done half a century earlier – could find no evidence that albumin was better than salt water. Since albumin is about 20 times more expensive than saline, huge sums of money from healthcare budgets worldwide must have been wasted over the past 50 years or so.

2. Design and conduct research properly

Stimulated by surveys revealing the poor quality of many reports of clinical trials, reporting standards have been developed and applied. Such standards make clear how many patients have been asked to participate in a study and how many declined the invitation. Results are presented according to the various treatment groups selected at the outset. But there is still a long way to go to improve: (a) the choice of questions being addressed in research; (b) the way that these questions are formulated to ensure that the outcomes of treatments chosen for assessment are those that patients regard as important; and (c) the information made available to patients. (See Chapters 11 and 12.)

To see whether a proposed trial might be feasible and acceptable, exploratory work involving groups of patients can be useful. This may highlight shortcomings in the design plans; or help to define outcomes that are more relevant; or even suggest that the concept is a non-starter.[5, 6]

This can save a lot of time, money, and frustration. The clinical trial in men with localized prostate cancer that we described in Chapter 11 (p140-141) showed how the research design was improved by careful consideration of the terms used by clinicians to describe the trial's purpose and the treatment options. Exploration of patients' views led to an acceptable study because the concerns and information needs of the men being invited to participate had been identified, and the information provided to potential participants took account of these findings.[7]

3. Publish all the results and make them accessible

Selective reporting of the results of research can lead to serious biases. Some 'negative' studies are never published when the results do not match the expectations of the investigators or funders. Without a published report to tell the tale, these trials disappear without trace.[8] Furthermore, results within published trials may be selectively reported – that is, some of the results are excluded because they are not so 'positive' for the treatment being tested.[9] Patients have suffered and died because of biased reporting of research on the effects of treatments. This practice is unethical as well as unscientific.

4. Produce unbiased and useful research reports

Even when studies are published, they often omit important elements that enable readers to assess and apply the findings. One review of 519 randomized trials published in reputable journals during December 2000 found that 82% did not describe the process of allocation concealment and 52% did not provide details of measures to reduce observer biases – both features that we suggested in Chapter 6 were crucial to good studies.[10] This poor reporting of details extends even to the description of the treatments used. A trial showing that giving a specific booklet (compared with no booklet) helped patients with irritable bowel syndrome, omitted to describe the contents of the booklet or how to obtain it; the 'treatment' could therefore not be used by any other patients or doctors. This was just one example in an analysis of trials in major journals that found about a third omit such crucial details.[11]

Finally, most published trials do not set their results in the context of previous similar trials. Without this key step, as we explained in Chapter 8, it is impossible to know what the results actually mean. Four-yearly checks of randomized trials reported in five major medical journals over a period of 12 years – 1997-2009 – illustrate the extent of the problem. Overall, only 25 of 94 (27%) reports made any reference at all to systematic reviews of similar trials. Only 3 of 94 reports actually contained updated reviews integrating the new results, and so showing what difference the new results had made to the totality of evidence. Sadly, there was no evidence of improvement in reporting practice with the passage of time.[12] This failure can lead to clinicians using different treatments depending on which journals they happen to read.

BLUEPRINT FOR A BETTER FUTURE

Medical research *could* be done for the right reasons and could be done and reported well. Taken individually, none of the suggestions that follows is novel. Taken together and promoted jointly by patients and clinicians, our eight action points constitute a blueprint for a better future in the testing and use of treatments.

1. Increase general knowledge about how to judge whether claims about treatment effects are trustworthy

A condition for change is greater public awareness of the ways in which bias and the play of chance can seriously distort evidence about the effects of treatments. One of the most important features of scientific investigation – recognizing and minimizing bias – can hardly be regarded as 'general knowledge' at present. We need more determined efforts to reduce these important gaps in understanding, and to make these concepts a routine part of education, from school age onwards.

2. Increase the capacity for preparing, maintaining, and disseminating systematic reviews of research evidence about the effects of treatments

Many of the answers to questions about the effects of treatments can be readily addressed by systematically reviewing evidence that already exists, by keeping such reviews up to date, and by disseminating the results efficiently to professionals and patients. There is a long way to go before the messages from existing evidence are readily available in systematic reviews. Addressing this deficiency should be one of the prime goals of health systems, so that reliable information about the effects of treatments is synthesized and made readily accessible.

3. Encourage honesty when there are uncertainties about the effects of treatments

Admitting uncertainty is often hard for health professionals, and it is sometimes not welcomed by patients. As a result, patients are sometimes given a false sense of security and are not informed about the uncertainties in the evidence. If clinicians and patients are to work together successfully for more efficient assessment of treatment effects, both must be more ready to acknowledge that inadequately evaluated treatments can do substantial harm; they must become more familiar with the methods needed to obtain reliable evidence. We need to find the best ways of making this happen.

4. Identify and prioritize research addressing questions deemed important by patients and clinicians

The portfolios of research funders and academic institutions are dominated by basic research that is unlikely to benefit patients in the foreseeable future, and by research directed at maximizing profits for industry. Applied research into questions that offer no potential to make money, yet matter to patients, has to fight for resources, even when it is publicly supported. We should see to it that more is done to identify what questions patients and clinicians are asking about the effects of treatments, and that research funders take account of them in prioritizing research to reduce these uncertainties.

5. Confront double standards on consent to treatment

Clinicians who are prepared to admit uncertainties about the effects of treatments and address them in formal treatment comparisons are subject to more stringent rules for interacting with patients than are their colleagues who are not. This perverse double standard is illogical and indefensible. When there are uncertainties about treatment effects, participation in randomized trials or other methods of unbiased evaluation should be the norm. We should ensure that participation in research on treatment effects is not presented as a necessarily risky endeavour, implying that 'standard' practice is always effective and safe.

6. Tackle inefficiencies within the research community

Many people are astonished to find that researchers are not required to assess systematically what is known already when they seek funding and ethical approval for new research. The consequence is inevitable – poorly designed and frankly unnecessary research continues on a scale that is unacceptable on ethical as well as scientific grounds. We should press research funders and research ethics committees to ensure that researchers do not embark on new research of any kind without referring to systematic reviews of existing relevant evidence. Reports of new research should begin by referring to systematic reviews showing why the additional research is needed, and end by showing what difference the new results have made to the totality of evidence.

7. Outlaw biased publication practices

To help stamp out biased publication practices steps are needed both when trials begin and when they end. When trials begin they should be registered and the protocols made publicly available for scrutiny. On completion, the results of all trials should be published and the raw data made accessible for scrutiny and further analysis.

8. Demand transparency of information about commercial and other conflicts of interests

There is now substantial evidence that vested financial and other interests sometimes take precedence over the interests of patients in the design, conduct, analysis, interpretation and use of research. This jeopardizes the mutual trust required to ensure that research serves the interests of patients more effectively. Everyone involved, from commercial companies to patient pressure groups, should be required to be transparent about any vested interests other than the well-being of patients.

Action is needed now

A revolution in testing treatments is long overdue. If professionals and patients act together, the steps that we advocate are eminently practicable. You, the readers, should demand change – now.

AN ACTION PLAN – THINGS YOU CAN DO

Identify questions about the effects of treatment that are important to you.

Learn to recognize uncertainty; speak up; ask questions; seek honest answers.

Don't be afraid to ask your doctor what treatments are available; what may happen if you choose a particular treatment; AND what might happen if you don't.

When thinking about possible treatments, you may find the information on decision aids at www.ohri.ca/DecisionAid helpful. See also: Additional Resources (Do you want to know more about shared decision-making?)

Use reliable websites such as NHS Choices (www.nhs.uk). See: Chapter 12 and the *Additional Resources* section in this book.

Be a healthy sceptic about unfounded claims and media reports of treatment 'breakthroughs'; about the way that 'numbers' are reported in the media – especially large numbers in headline claims!

Challenge treatments offered to you or your family on the basis of beliefs and dogmas, but unsubstantiated by reliable evidence.

Be wary of unnecessary disease 'labelling' and over-investigation (see Chapters 2 and 4) – find out if the disease in question is considered high risk or low risk for you. Ask what would happen if nothing immediate is done.

Agree to participate in a clinical trial only on condition (i) that the study protocol has been registered and made publicly available (ii) that the protocol refers to systematic reviews of existing evidence showing that the trial is justified; and (iii) that you receive a written assurance that the full study results will be published, and sent to all participants who indicate that they wish to receive them.

Encourage and work with health professionals, researchers, research funders, and others who are trying to promote research addressing inadequately answered questions about the effects of treatment which you regard as important.

Encourage wider education about the effects of biases and the play of chance, and lobby your elected political representative and others about doing more to emphasize this in school curricula, beginning in primary schools.

References

Foreword Ben Goldacre

1   Lexchin J, Bero LA, Djulbegovic B, *et al*. Pharmaceutical industry sponsorship and research outcome and quality: systematic review. *BMJ* 2003; 326:1167-70.

2   Schwitzer G, Ganapati M, Henry D, *et al*. What are the roles and responsibilities of the media in disseminating health information? *PLoS Med* 2(7):e215.

3   Wilson PM, Booth AM, Eastwood A, et al. Deconstructing media coverage of trastuzumab (Herceptin): an analysis of national newspaper coverage. *Journal of the Royal Society of Medicine* 2008;101:125-32.

4   Shang A, Huwiler-Müntener K, Nartey L, *et al*. Are the clinical effects of homoeopathy placebo effects? Comparative study of placebo-controlled trials of homoeopathy and allopathy. *Lancet* 2005;366:726-32.

5   Bjelakovic G, Nikolova D, Gluud LL, et al. Antioxidant supplements for prevention of mortality in healthy participants and patients with various diseases. *Cochrane Database of Systematic Reviews* 2008, Issue 2. Art. No.: CD007176.

Introduction

1   Nolte E, McKee CM. *Does health care save lives? Avoidable mortality revisited.* London: Nuffield Trust, 2004.

2   Nolte E, McKee CM. Measuring the health of nations: updating an earlier analysis. *Health Affairs* 2008;27(1): 58-77.

3   Gigerenzer G. *Reckoning with risk.* London: Penguin Books, 2003. Citing Franklin B. Letter to Jean Baptiste Le Roy, 13 November 1789. Writings, vol x.

4   Goldacre B. *Bad Science.* London: Fourth Estate, 2008, px.

5   Matthews A, Dowswell T, Haas DM, *et al*. Interventions for nausea and vomiting in early pregnancy. *Cochrane Database of Systematic Reviews* 2010, Issue 9. Art. No.: CD007575.

6   Irwig L, Irwig J, Trevena L, *et al*. Smart health choices: making sense of health advice. London: Hammersmith Press, 2008. pdf freely available at: www.health.usyd.edu.au/shdg/resources/smart_health_choices.php and from www.jameslindlibrary.org.

7   Woloshin S, Schwartz LM, Welch HG. *Know your chances: understanding health statistics.* Berkeley: University of California Press, 2008. pdf freely available at www.jameslindlibrary.org.

Chapter 1. New – but is it better?

1   Vandenbroucke JP. Thalidomide: an unanticipated adverse event. 2003. Available from: www.jameslindlibrary.org.

2   Stephens T, Brynner R. *Dark medicine: the impact of thalidomide and its revival as a vital medicine.* Cambridge, Mass: Perseus Publishing, 2001.

3   Thomson D, Capstick T. How a risk management programme can ensure safety in thalidomide use. *Pharmaceutical Journal* 2004 Feb 14:194-5.

4   Krumholz HM, Ross JR, Presler AH, *et al.* What have we learnt from Vioxx? *BMJ* 2007;334:120-3.

5   Merck statements dated 7 December 2009, on Vioxx proceedings in Ontario, Canada, and 4 March 2010 on Vioxx judgment in Australia, available at www.merck.com.

6   Cohen D. Rosiglitazone what went wrong? *BMJ* 2010;341:c4848.

7   Lehman R, Yudkin JS, Krumholz HM. Licensing drugs for diabetes: surrogate end points are not enough, robust evidence of benefits and harms is needed. *BMJ* 2010;341:c4805.

8   Blackstone EH. Could it happen again? The Björk-Shiley convexo-concave heart valve story. *Circulation* 2005;111:2717-19.

9   Wilson PM, Booth AM, Eastwood A, *et al.* Deconstructing media coverage of trastuzumab (Herceptin): an analysis of national newspaper coverage. *Journal of the Royal Society of Medicine* 2008;101:125-32.

10 Timmins N. Drugs watchdog gets harsh treatment. *Financial Times,* 8 October 2005, p6.

11 Hawkes N. Wonder drug is "cure" for cancer, say doctors. *The Times,* 20 October 2005.

12 Press MF, Sauter G, Bernstein L, *et al.* Diagnostic evaluation of HER-2 as a molecular target: an assessment of accuracy and reproducibility of laboratory testing in large, prospective, randomized clinical trials. *Clinical Cancer Research* 2005;11(18):6598-607.

13 NICE draft guidance on trastuzumab (Herceptin) for early breast cancer (press release), 9 June 2006. www.nice.org.uk/page.aspx?o=328789.

14 Cumming J, Mays N, Daubé J. How New Zealand has contained expenditure on drugs. *BMJ* 2010;340:1224-6.

15 NHS NICE Technology Appraisal TA34. *Guidance on the use of trastuzumab for the treatment of advanced breast cancer.* Issue date March 2002; review date April 2005. www.nice.org.uk/TA34.

Chapter 2. Hoped-for effects that don't materialize

1   Gilbert R, Salanti G, Harden M, *et al.* Infant sleeping position and the sudden infant death syndrome: systematic review of observational studies and historical review of clinicians' recommendations from 1940-2000. *International Journal of Epidemiology* 2005;34:74-87.

2   Furberg CD. Effect of antiarrhythmic drugs on mortality after myocardial infarction. *American Journal of Cardiology* 1983;52:32C-36C.

3   Chalmers I. In the dark. Drug companies should be forced to publish all the results of clinical trials. How else can we know the truth about their products? *New Scientist* 2004, 6 March, p19. Citing Moore T, *Deadly Medicine.* New York: Simon and Schuster, 1995.

4   Cowley AJ, Skene A, Stainer K, *et al.* The effect of lorcainide on arrhythmias and survival in patients with acute myocardial infarction: an example of publication bias. *International Journal of Cardiology* 1993;40:161-6.

5   Chalmers I. Evaluating the effects of care during pregnancy and childbirth. In: Chalmers I, Enkin M, Keirse MJNC, eds. *Effective care in pregnancy and*

childbirth. Oxford: Oxford University Press, 1989:3-38.

6 Ulfelder H. The stilbestrol disorders in historical perspective. *Cancer* 1980;45:3008-11.

7 Office of Technology Assessment. *Identifying health technologies that work: searching for evidence.* Washington, DC: US Government Printing Office, 1994.

8 Hemminki E, McPherson K. Impact of postmenopausal hormone therapy on cardiovascular events and cancer: pooled data from clinical trials. *BMJ* 1997;315:149-53.

9 Anonymous. HRT: update on the risk of breast cancer and long-term safety. *Current Problems in Pharmacovigilance* 2003;29:1-3. Citing results of Women's Health Initiative randomized controlled trial (*JAMA* 2003;289:3243-53) and Million Women Study (*Lancet* 2003;362:419-27).

10 Roberts H. Hormone replacement therapy comes full circle. *BMJ* 2007;335:219-20.

11 Williams HC. Evening primrose oil for atopic dermatitis: time to say goodnight (editorial). *BMJ* 2003;327:1358-9.

12 Hoare C, Li Wan Po A, Williams H. Systematic review of treatment for atopic eczema. *Health Technology Assessment* 2000;4(37):1-191.

13 Takwale A, Tan E, Agarwal S, *et al.* Efficacy and tolerability of borage oil in adults and children with atopic eczema: randomised, double blind, placebo controlled, parallel group trial. *BMJ* 2003;327:1385-7.

Chapter 3. More is not necessarily better

1 Crile G. A plea against blind fear of cancer. *Life*, 31 October 1955, pp128-32.

2 Baum M, Houghton J. Contribution of randomised controlled trials to understanding and management of early breast cancer. *BMJ* 1999;319:568-71.

3 Veronesi U, Cascinelli N, Mariani L, *et al.* Twenty-year follow up of a randomized study comparing breast-conserving surgery with radical mastectomy for early breast cancer. *New England Journal of Medicine* 2002;347:1227-32.

4 Baum M. *Breast beating: a personal odyssey in the quest for an understanding of breast cancer, the meaning of life and other easy questions.* London: Anshan, 2010.

5 Japanese Breast Cancer Society. Results of questionnaires concerning breast cancer surgery in Japan 1980-2003. *Breast Cancer* 2005;12(1).

6 Early Breast Cancer Trialists' Collaborative Group. Effects of adjuvant tamoxifen and of cytotoxic therapy on mortality in early breast cancer. An overview of 61 randomized trials among 28,896 women. *New England Journal of Medicine* 1988;319:1681-92.

7 Clinical Trial Service Unit website: www.ctsu.ox.ac.uk.

8 The Cochrane Collaboration website: www.cochrane.org.

9 Kolata G, Eichenwald K. Health business thrives on unproven treatment, leaving science behind. *New York Times* Special Report, 2 October 1999.

10 Farquhar C, Marjoribanks J, Basser R, *et al.* High dose chemotherapy and autologous bone marrow or stem cell transplantation versus conventional chemotherapy for women with early poor prognosis breast cancer. *Cochrane Database of Systematic Reviews* 2005, Issue 3. Art. No.:

CD003139.

11 Farquhar C, Marjoribanks J, Basser R, *et al.* High dose chemotherapy and autologous bone marrow or stem cell transplantation versus conventional chemotherapy for women with metastatic breast cancer. *Cochrane Database of Systematic Reviews* 2005, Issue 3. Art. No.: CD003142.

12 Piccart-Gebhart MJ, Procter M, Leyland-Jones B, *et al.* Trastuzumab after adjuvant chemotherapy in HER-2-positive breast cancer. *New England Journal of Medicine* 2005;353:1659-72.

13 Romond EH, Perez EA, Bryant J, *et al.* Trastuzumab plus adjuvant chemotherapy for operable HER-2-positive breast cancer. *New England Journal of Medicine* 2005;353:1673-84.

14 Carlson GW, Woods WC. Management of axillary lymph node metastasis in breast cancer: making progress. *JAMA* 2011;305:606-7.

Chapter 4. Earlier is not necessarily better

1 Raffle A, Gray M. *Screening: evidence and practice.* Oxford: Oxford University Press, rev. repr., 2009.

2 Sense About Science. *Making sense of screening.* London: Sense About Science, 2009. Available from www.senseaboutscience.org.

3 Goodman MT, Gurney JG, Smith MA, *et al.* Sympathetic nervous system tumors. In: Ries LAG, Smith MA, Gurney JG, *et al* (eds). *Cancer incidence and survival among children and adolescents: United States SEER Program 1975-1995.* National Cancer Institute, SEER Program. NIH Pub. No.99-4649. Bethesda, MD, 1999. SEER Pediatric Monograph available at http://seer.cancer.gov/publications/childhood.

4 Mullassery D, Dominici C, Jesudason EC, *et al.* Neuroblastoma: contemporary management. *Archives of Disease in Childhood – Education and Practice* 2009;94:177-85.

5 Morris JK. Screening for neuroblastoma in children. *Journal of Medical Screening* 2002;9:56.

6 Raffle A, Gray M. *op. cit.,* pp89-92.

7 Welch HG. *Should I be tested for cancer? Maybe not and here's why.* Berkeley and Los Angeles: University of California Press, 2004, p77.

8 Cosford PA, Leng GC, Thomas J. Screening for abdominal aortic aneurysm. *Cochrane Database of Systematic Reviews*, 2007, Issue 2, Art. No.: CD002945.

9 Welch HG. Screening mammography – a long run for a short slide? *New England Journal of Medicine* 2010; 363:1276-8.

10 Heath I. It is not wrong to say no. Why are women told only the benefits of breast screening and none of the possible harms? *BMJ* 2009; 338:1534.

11 Gøtzsche PC, Nielsen M. Screening for breast cancer with mammography. *Cochrane Database of Systematic Reviews* 2011, Issue 1. Art. No.: CD001877.

12 Kösters JP, Gøtzsche PC. Regular self-examination or clinical examination for early detection of breast cancer. *Cochrane Database of Systematic Reviews* 2003, Issue 2. Art. No.: CD003373. (No change, Update, Issue 3, July 2008.)

13 McPherson K. Should we screen for breast cancer? *BMJ* 2010:340:c3106.

14 Cancer Research UK. Prostate cancer – UK incidence statistics. Updated 23 December 2010. http://info.cancerresearchuk.org/cancerstats/types/

prostate/incidence.

15 Chapman S, Barratt A, Stockler M. *Let sleeping dogs lie? What men should know before getting tested for prostate cancer.* Sydney: Sydney University Press, 2010. pdf available from: http://ses.library.usyd.edu.au/bitstream/2123/6835/3/Let-sleeping-dogs-lie.pdf.

16 Holmström B, Johansson M, Bergh A, *et al.* Prostate specific antigen for early detection of prostate cancer: longitudinal study. *BMJ* 2009;339:b3537.

17 Djulbegovic M, Beyth RJ, Neuberger MM, *et al.* Screening for prostate cancer: systematic review and meta-analysis of randomised controlled trials. *BMJ* 2010;341:c4543.

18 Stark JR, Mucci L, Rothman KJ, *et al.* Prostate cancer screening: the controversy continues. *BMJ* 2009;339:b3601.

19 National Lung Screening Trial Research Team. Reduced lung-cancer mortality with low-dose computed tomographic screening. *New England Journal of Medicine* 2011;365:395-409.

20 Moynihan R. Beware the fortune tellers peddling genetic tests. *BMJ* 2010;341:c7233.

21 Thornton H. The screening debates: time for a broader approach? *European Journal of Cancer* 2003;39:1807-9.

22 Adapted from Wilson JMG, Jungner G. *Principles and practice of screening for disease.* Public health paper no 34. Geneva: World Health Organization, 1968.

23 COMARE 12th Report: The impact of personally initiated X-ray computed tomography scanning for the health assessment of asymptomatic individuals. Press release, 19 December 2007. www.comare.org.uk/12thReportPressRelease.htm.

24 Department of Health. Better protection for patients having 'MOT' scans: http://webarchive.nationalarchives.gov.uk/+/www.dh.gov.uk/en/MediaCentre/Pressreleasesarchive/DH_115243.

25 Food and Drug Administration. Radiation-emitting products: Computed tomography and full-body CT scans – what you need to know: www.fda.gov/radiation-emittingProducts.

Chapter 5. Dealing with uncertainty about the effects of treatments

1 Cabello JB, Burls A. Emparanza JI, *et al.* Oxygen therapy for acute myocardial infarction. *Cochrane Database of Systematic Reviews* 2010, Issue 6. Art No.: CD007160.

2 Glasziou P, Chalmers I, Rawlins M, *et al.* When are randomised trials unnecessary? Picking signal from noise. *BMJ* 2007;334:349-51.

3 Goh CL. Flashlamp-pumped pulsed dye laser (585nm) for the treatment of portwine stains: a study of treatment outcome in 94 Asian patients in Singapore. *Singapore Medical Journal* 2000;41:24-28.

4 Druker BJ, Talpaz M, Resta DJ, *et al.* Efficacy and safety of a specific inhibitor of the BCR-ABL tyrosine kinase in chronic myeloid leukemia. *New England Journal of Medicine* 2001;344:1031-7.

5 Goldman J for the British Committee for Standards in Haematology. *Recommendations for the management of BCR-ABL-positive chronic myeloid leukaemia.* London: BSH, 2007.

6 Purohit N, Ray S, Wilson T, *et al.* The parent's kiss: an effective way to remove paediatric nasal foreign bodies. *Annals of the Royal College of*

Surgeons of England 2008:90:420-2.

7 Sanghavi DM. How should we tell the stories of our medical miracles? *Lancet* 2010;375:2068-9.

8 Léauté-Labrèze C, Dumas la Roque E, Hubische T, *et al.* Propranolol for severe hemangiomas of infancy. *New England Journal of Medicine* 2008;358:2649-51.

9 Huikeshoven M, Koster PHL, de Borgie CAJM, *et al.* Re-darkening of port-wine stains 10 years after pulsed-dye-laser treatment. *New England Journal of Medicine* 2007;356:1235-40.

10 Waner M. Recent developments in lasers and the treatment of birthmarks. *Archives of Disease in Childhood* 2003;88:372-4.

11 Anti-Thrombotic Trialists' (ATT) Collaboration. Clinical Trial Service Unit website: www.ctsu.ox.ac.uk/projects/att.

12 Lin CWC, Moseley AM, Refshauge KM. Rehabilitation for ankle fractures in adults. *Cochrane Database of Systematic Reviews* 2008, Issue 3. Art. No.: CD005595.

13 Lindley RI. Personal communication, 2005.

14 Wardlaw JM, Murray V, Berge E, *et al.* Thrombolysis for acute ischaemic stroke. *Cochrane Database of Systematic Reviews* 2009, Issue 4. Art. No.: CD000213.

15 Schmidt B, Roberts RS, Davis P, *et al*; for the Caffeine for Apnea of Prematurity Trial Group. Long-term effects of caffeine therapy for apnea of prematurity. *New England Journal of Medicine* 2007;357:1893-902.

16 Caffeine citrate (Comment) in *Neonatal Formulary 5*. Available from: www.blackwellpublishing.com/medicine/bmj/nnf5/pdfs/comment/caffeine1.pdf.

17 Kenyon S, Pike, K, Jones DR, *et al.* Childhood outcomes after prescription of antibiotics to pregnant women with preterm rupture of the membranes: 7-year follow-up of the ORACLE I trial. *Lancet* 2008;372:1310-18.

18 Kenyon S, Pike K, Jones DR, *et al.* Childhood outcomes after prescription of antibiotics to pregnant women with spontaneous preterm labour: 7-year follow-up of the ORACLE II trial. *Lancet* 2008;372:1319-27.

19 Erythromycin (Comment) in: *Neonatal Formulary 5*. Available from: www.blackwellpublishing.com/medicine/bmj/nnf5/pdfs/commentary/erythromycin.pdf.

20 Giuliano AE, Hunt KK, Ballman KV, *et al.* Axillary dissection vs no axillary dissection in women with invasive breast cancer and sentinel node metastasis: a randomized clinical trial. *JAMA* 2011;305:569-75.

21 General Medical Council. *Good Medical Practice*. London: GMC, 2006, p13.

22 Ashcroft R. Giving medicine a fair trial. *BMJ* 2000;320:1686.

23 Pritchard-Jones K, Dixon-Woods M, Naafs-Wilstra M, *et al.* Improving recruitment to clinical trials for cancer in childhood. *Lancet Oncology* 2008;9:392-9.

24 Equator network resource centre for good reporting of health research studies: www.equator-network.org.

25 Smithells RW. Iatrogenic hazards and their effects. *Postgraduate Medical Journal* 1975;15:39-52.

Chapter 6. Fair tests of treatments

1 Hopkins WA. Patulin in the common cold. IV. Biological properties: extended trial in the common cold. *Lancet* 1943;ii:631-5.

2 Sanders TAB, Woolfe R, Rantzen E. Controlled evaluation of slimming diets: use of television for recruitment. *Lancet* 1990;336:918-20.

3 Glasziou P, Chalmers I, Rawlins M, *et al*. When are randomised trials unnecessary? Picking signal from noise. *BMJ* 2007;334: 349-51.

4 Pocock SJ. Randomised clinical trials. *BMJ* 1977;1:1661.

5 Balfour TG. Quoted in West C (1854). *Lectures on the Diseases of Infancy and Childhood*. London: Longman, Brown, Green and Longmans, p600.

6 King G, Gakidou E, Imai K, *et al*. Public policy for the poor? A randomised assessment of the Mexican universal health insurance programme. *Lancet* 2009;373:1447-54.

7 Peto J, Eden OB, Lilleyman J, *et al*. Improvement in treatments for children with acute lymphoblastic leukaemia: The Medical Research Council UKALL Trials, 1972-84. *Lancet* 1986;i:408-11.

8 Noseworthy JH, Ebers GC, Vandervoort MK, *et al*. The impact of blinding on the results of a randomized, placebo-controlled multiple sclerosis clinical trial. *Neurology* 1994;44:16-20.

9 Moseley JB, O'Malley K, Petersen NJ, *et al*. A controlled trial of arthroscopic surgery for osteoarthritis of the knee. *New England Journal of Medicine* 2002;347:81-8.

10 Venning GR. Validity of anecdotal reports of suspected adverse drug reactions: the problem of false alarms. *BMJ* 1982;284:249-54.

11 McLernon DJ, Bond CM, Hannaford PC, *et al* on behalf of the Yellow Card Collaborative. Adverse drug reaction reporting in the UK: a retrospective observational comparison of Yellow Card reports submitted by patients and healthcare professionals. *Drug Safety* 2010;33:775-88.

12 Kocher T. Ueber Kropfexstirpation und ihre Folgen. *Archiv für Klinische Chirurgie* 1883;29:254-337.

13 Silverman WA, Andersen DH, Blanc WA, *et al*. A difference in mortality rate and incidence of kernicterus among premature infants allotted to two prophylactic regimens. *Pediatrics* 1956;18:614-25.

14 Zhang J, Ding E, Song Y. Adverse effects of cyclooxygenase 2 inhibitors on renal and arrhythmia events: meta-analysis of randomized trials. *JAMA* 2006;296:1619-21.

15 Vandenbroucke JP, Psaty BM. Benefits and risks of drug treatments: how to combine the best evidence on benefits with the best data about adverse effects. *JAMA* 2008;300:2417-9.

16 Whittington CJ, Kendall T, Fonagy P, *et al*. Selective serotonin reuptake inhibitors in childhood depression: systematic review of published versus unpublished data. *Lancet* 2004;363:1341-5.

Chapter 7. Taking account of the play of chance

1 Antithrombotic Trialists' (ATT) Collaboration. Aspirin in the primary and secondary prevention of vascular disease: collaborative meta-analysis of individual participant data from randomised trials. *Lancet* 2009;373:1849-60.

2 CRASH trial collaborators. Final results of MRC CRASH, a randomised placebo-controlled trial of intravenous corticosteroid in adults with head injury – outcomes at 6 months. *Lancet* 2005;365:1957-9.

3 CRASH-2 trial collaborators. Effects of tranexamic acid on death, vascular occlusive events, and blood transfusion in trauma patients with significant

haemorrhage (CRASH-2): a randomised, placebo-controlled trial. *Lancet* 2010;376:23-32.

4 Askie LM, Brocklehurst P, Darlow BA, *et al* and the NeOProM Collaborative Group. NeOProM: Neonatal Oxygenation Prospective Meta-analysis Collaboration study protocol. *BMC Pediatrics* 2011; 11:6.

Chapter 8. Assessing all the relevant, reliable evidence
1 ISIS-2 (Second International Study of Infarct Survival) Collaborative Group. Randomised trial of intravenous streptokinase, oral aspirin, both, or neither among 17,187 cases of suspected acute myocardial infarction: ISIS-2. *Lancet* 1988;332:349-60.

2 Reynolds LA, Tansey EM, eds. *Prenatal corticosteroids for reducing morbidity and mortality after preterm birth*. London: Wellcome Trust Centre for the History of Medicine, 2005.

3 Dickersin K, Chalmers I. Recognising, investigating and dealing with incomplete and biased reporting of clinical research: from Francis Bacon to the World Health Organisation. James Lind Library 2010 (www.jameslindlibrary.org).

4 Cowley AJ, Skene A, Stainer K, *et al*. The effect of lorcainide on arrhythmias and survival in patients with acute myocardial infarction: an example of publication bias. *International Journal of Cardiology* 1993;40:161-6.

5 Moore T. *Deadly Medicine*. New York: Simon and Schuster, 1995.

6 Stjernswärd J. Decreased survival related to irradiation postoperatively in early operable breast cancer. *Lancet* 1974;ii:1285-6.

7 Stjernswärd J. Meta-analysis as a manifestation of 'bondförnuft' ('peasant sense'). JLL Bulletin: Commentaries on the history of treatment evaluation 2009 (www.jameslindlibrary.org).

8 Fugh-Berman AJ. The haunting of medical journals: how ghostwriting sold "HRT". *PLoS Medicine* 2010;7(9):e1000335.

9 Whittington CJ, Kendall T, Fonagy P, *et al*. Selective serotonin-reuptake inhibitors in childhood depression: systematic review of published versus unpublished data. *Lancet* 2004;363:1341-5.

10 Spielmans GI, Biehn TL, Sawrey DL. A case study of salami slicing: pooled analysis of duloxetine for depression. *Psychotherapy and Psychosomatics* 2010;79:97-106.

11 Antman EM, Lau J, Kupelnick B, *et al*. A comparison of results of meta-analysis of randomized control trials and recommendations of clinical experts. *JAMA* 1992;268:240-8.

12 Natanson C, Kern SJ, Lurie P, *et al*. Cell-free hemoglobin-based blood substitutes and risk of myocardial infarction and death: a meta-analysis. *JAMA* 2008;299(19):2304-12.

13 Chalmers I. TGN1412 and *The Lancet*'s solicitation of reports of phase 1 trials. *Lancet* 2006;368:2206-7.

14 Jack A. Call to release human drug trial data. *Financial Times*, 8 August 2006.

15 Kenter MJH, Cohen AF. Establishing risk of human experimentation with drugs: lessons from TGN1412. *Lancet* 2006;368:1387-91.

16 McLellan F. 1966 and all that – when is a literature search done? *Lancet* 2001;358:646.

17 Horn J, Limburg M. Calcium antagonists for acute ischemic stroke.

Cochrane Database of Systematic Reviews 2000, Issue 1. Art. No.: CD001928.

18 Horn J, de Haan RJ, Vermeulen M, *et al.* Nimodipine in animal model experiments of focal cerebral ischemia: a systematic review. *Stroke* 2001;32:2433-8.

19 O'Collins VE, Macleod MR, Donnan GA, *et al.* 1,026 experimental treatments in acute stroke. *Annals of Neurology* 2006;59:467-77.

20 CRASH trial collaborators. Final results of MRC CRASH, a randomised placebo-controlled trial of intravenous corticosteroid in adults with head injury – outcomes at 6 months. *Lancet* 2005;365:1957-9.

Chapter 9. Regulating tests of treatments: help or hindrance?

1 Emanuel EJ, Menikoff J. Reforming the regulations governing research with human subjects. *New England Journal of Medicine* 2011;10.1056/ NEJMsb1106942.NEJM.org.

2 Chalmers I, Lindley R. Double standards on informed consent to treatment. In: Doyal L, Tobias JS, eds. *Informed consent in medical research.* London: BMJ Books 2001, pp266-75.

3 Fallowfield L, Jenkins V, Farewell V, *et al.* Efficacy of a Cancer Research UK communicating skills training model for oncologists: a randomised controlled trial. *Lancet* 2002;359:650-6.

4 Chalmers I. Regulation of therapeutic research is compromising the interests of patients. *International Journal of Pharmaceutical Medicine* 2007;21:395-404.

5 Roberts I, Prieto-Marino D, Shakur H, *et al.* Effect of consent rituals on mortality in emergency care research. *Lancet* 2011;377:1071-2.

Chapter 10. Research – good, bad, and unnecessary

1 Equator network resource centre for good reporting of health research studies: www.equator-network.org.

2 European Carotid Surgery Trialists' Collaborative Group. Randomised trial of endarterectomy for recently symptomatic carotid stenosis: final results of the MRC European Carotid Surgery Trial (ECST). *Lancet* 1998;351:1379-87.

3 Cina CS, Clase CM, Haynes RB. Carotid endarterectomy for symptomatic carotid stenosis. *The Cochrane Database of Systematic Reviews* 1999, Issue 3. Art. No.: CD001081.

4 The Magpie Trial Collaborative Group. Do women with pre-eclampsia, and their babies, benefit from magnesium sulphate? The Magpie Trial: a randomised, placebo-controlled trial. *Lancet* 2002;359:1877-90.

5 Duley L, Gülmezoglu AM, Henderson-Smart DJ. Magnesium sulphate and other anticonvulsants for women with pre-eclampsia. *Cochrane Database of Systematic Reviews* 2003, Issue 2. Art. No.: CD000025.

6 Global Report. UNAIDS report on the Global AIDS epidemic 2010: www. unaids.org/globalreport/Global_report.htm.

7 Grimwade K, Swingler G. Cotrimoxazole prophylaxis for opportunistic infections in adults with HIV. *Cochrane Database of Systematic Reviews* 2003, Issue 3. Art. No.: CD003108.

8 Chintu C, Bhat GJ, Walker AS, *et al.* Co-trimoxazole as prophylaxis against opportunistic infections in HIV-infected Zambian children (CHAP): a double blind randomised placebo-controlled trial. *Lancet* 2004;364:1865-

71.

9 MRC News Release. Antibiotic drug almost halves AIDS-related death in children. London: MRC, 19 November 2004.

10 World Health Organization and UNICEF. *Co-trimoxazole prophylaxis for HIV-exposed and HIV-infected infants and children: practical approaches to implementation and scale up.* WHO and UNICEF, 2009.

11 Soares K, McGrath J, Adams C. Evidence and tardive dyskinesia. *Lancet* 1996;347:1696-7.

12 Thornley B, Adams C. Content and quality of 2000 controlled trials in schizophrenia over 50 years. *BMJ* 1998;317:1181-4.

13 Howell CJ, Chalmers I. A review of prospectively controlled comparisons of epidural with non-epidural forms of pain relief during labour. *International Journal of Obstetric Anesthesia* 1992;1:93-110.

14 Horn J, Limburg M. Calcium antagonists for acute ischemic stroke. *Cochrane Database of Systematic Reviews* 2000, Issue 1. Art No.: CD001928.

15 Horn J, de Haan RJ, Vermeulen RD, Luiten PGM, *et al*. Nimodipine in animal model experiments of focal cerebral ischemia: a systematic review. *Stroke* 2001;32:2433-8.

16 Fergusson D, Glass KC, Hutton B, *et al*. Randomized controlled trials of aprotinin in cardiac surgery: using clinical equipoise to stop the bleeding. *Clinical Trials* 2005;2:218-32.

17 Tallon D, Chard J, Dieppe P. Relation between agendas of the research community and the research consumer. *Lancet* 2000;355:2037-40.

18 Cream J, Cayton H. New drugs for Alzheimer's disease – a consumer perspective. *CPD Bulletin Old Age Psychiatry* 2001;2:80-2.

19 Cohen CI, D'Onofrio A, Larkin L, *et al*. A comparison of consumer and provider preferences for research on homeless veterans. *Community Mental Health Journal* 1999;35:273-9.

20 Griffiths KM, Jorm AF, Christensen H, *et al*. Research priorities in mental health, Part 2: an evaluation of the current research effort against stakeholders' priorities. *Australian and New Zealand Journal of Psychiatry* 2002;36:327-39.

21 Oliver S, Gray J. *A bibliography of research reports about patients', clinicians' and researchers' priorities for new research.* London: James Lind Alliance, December, 2006.

22 Chalmers I. Current controlled trials: an opportunity to help improve the quality of clinical research. *Current Controlled Trials in Cardiovascular Medicine* 2000;1:3-8. Available from: http://cvm.controlled-trials.com/content/1/1/3.

23 Editorial. Safeguarding participants in controlled trials. *Lancet* 2000;355:1455-63.

24 Fugh-Berman A. The haunting of medical journals: how ghostwriting sold "HRT". *PLoS Medicine* 2010:7(9):e10000335.

25 Heimans L, van Hylckama V, Dekker FW. Are claims of advertisements in medical journals supported by RCTs? *Netherlands Journal of Medicine* 2010;68:46-9.

26 Lexchin J, Bero LA, Djulbeovic B, *et al*. Pharmaceutical industry sponsorship and research outcome and quality: systematic review. *BMJ* 2003;326:1167-76.

27 Weatherall D. Academia and industry: increasingly uneasy bedfellows.

Lancet 2000;355:1574.

28 Angell M. Is academic medicine for sale? *New England Journal of Medicine* 2000;342:1516-8.

29 Grant J, Green L, Mason B. From bench to bedside: Comroe and Dripps revisited. HERG Research Report No. 30. Uxbridge, Middlesex: Brunel University Health Economics Research Group, 2003.

30 Pound P, Ebrahim S, Sandercock P, *et al.* Reviewing Animal Trials Systematically (RATS) Group. Where is the evidence that animal research benefits humans? *BMJ* 2004;328:514-7.

31 Weatherall D. The quiet art revisited. *Lancet* 2011;377:1912-13.

32 Pirmohamed M. Cited in Mayor S. Fitting the drug to the patient. *BMJ* 2007;334:452-3.

33 Editorial. The human genome at ten. *Nature* 2010;464:649-50.

34 Mackillop WJ, Palmer MJ, O'Sullivan B, *et al.* Clinical trials in cancer: the role of surrogate patients in defining what constitutes an ethically acceptable clinical experiment. *British Journal of Cancer* 1989;59:388-95.

35 The Psoriasis Association: www.psoriasis-association.org.uk.

36 National Psoriasis Association. Statistics about psoriasis: www.psoriasis. org/netcommunity/learn_statistics.

37 Jobling R. Therapeutic research into psoriasis: patients' perspectives, priorities and interests. In: Rawlins M, Littlejohns P, ed. *Delivering quality in the NHS 2005*. Abingdon: Radcliffe Publishing Ltd, pp53-6.

Chapter 11. Getting the right research done is everybody's business

1 Oliver S, Clarke-Jones L, Rees R, *et al.* Involving consumers in research and development agenda setting for the NHS: developing an evidence-based approach. *Health Technology Assessment Report* 2004;8(15).

2 NIHR Guy's and St. Thomas' and King's College London's Biomedical Research Centre. *Involving users in the research process: a 'how to' guide for researchers*. Version 1, April 2010. Available from: www. biomedicalresearchcentre.org.

3 Cartwright J, Crowe S. *Patient and public involvement toolkit*. London: Wiley-Blackwell and BMJI Books, 2011.

4 European Science Foundation/EMRC. *Implementation of medical research in clinical practice – a growing challenge*. Strasbourg: ESF, 2011.

5 Hanley B, Truesdale A, King A, *et al.* Involving consumers in designing, conducting, and interpreting randomised controlled trials: questionnaire survey. *BMJ* 2001;322:519-23.

6 Koops L, Lindley RI. Thrombolysis for acute ischaemic stroke: consumer involvement in design of new randomised controlled trial. *BMJ* 2002;325:415-7.

7 Staley K. *Exploring impact: public involvement in NHS, public health and social care research*. Eastleigh: INVOLVE, 2009. Available from: www.invo. org.uk.

8 Petit-Zeman S, Firkins L, Scadding JW. The James Lind Alliance: tackling research mismatches. *Lancet* 2010;376:667-9.

9 Patient Partner Project. An EU programme 'Identifying the needs for patients partnering in clinical research': www.patientpartner-europe.eu.

10 Thornton H, Edwards A, Elwyn G. Evolving the multiple roles of 'patients' in health-care research: reflections after involvement in a trial of shared

decision-making. *Health Expectations* 2003;6:189-97.

11 Dixon-Woods M, Agarwal S, Young B *et al.* Integrative approaches to qualitative and quantitative evidence. NHS Health Development Agency, 2004.

12 Kushner R. *Breast cancer: a personal history and an investigative report.* New York: Harcourt Brace Jovanovitch, 1975.

13 Lerner BH. *The breast cancer wars: hope, fear, and the pursuit of a cure in twentieth-century America.* New York: Oxford University Press, 2003.

14 Institute of Medical Ethics Working Party on the ethical implications of AIDS: AIDS, ethics, and clinical trials. *BMJ* 1992;305:699-701.

15 Thornton H. The patient's role in research. [Paper given at *The Lancet* 'Challenge of Breast Cancer' Conference, Brugge, April 1994.] In: Health Committee Third Report. *Breast cancer services. Volume II. Minutes of evidence and appendices.* London: HMSO, July 1995, 112-4.

16 Concorde Coordinating Committee. Concorde: MRC/ANRS randomised double-blind controlled trial of immediate and deferred zidovudine in symptom-free HIV infection. *Lancet* 1994;343:871-81.

17 Perehudoff K, Alves TL. *Patient and consumer organisations at the European Medicines Agency: financial disclosure and transparency.* Amsterdam: Health Action International, 2010. Available from www.haieurope.org.

18 Herxheimer A. Relationships between the pharmaceutical industry and patients' organisations. *BMJ* 2003;326:1208-10.

19 Consumers' Association. Who's injecting the cash? *Which?* 2003, April, pp24-25.

20 Koops L, Lindley RI. Thrombolysis for acute ischaemic stroke: consumer involvement in design of new randomised controlled trial. *BMJ* 2002;325:415-7.

21 Donovan J, Mills N, Smith M, *et al* for the ProtecT Study Group. Quality improvement report: improving design and conduct of randomised trials by embedding them in qualitative research: ProtecT (prostate testing for cancer and treatment) study. *BMJ* 2002;325:766-70.

Chapter 12. So what makes for better healthcare?

1 Edwards A, Elwyn G, Atwell C, *et al.* Shared decision making and risk communication in general practice – a study incorporating systematic literature reviews, psychometric evaluation of outcome measures, and quantitative, qualitative and health economic analyses of a cluster randomised trial of professional skill development. Report to Health in Partnership programme, UK Department of Health. Cardiff: Department of General Practice. University of Wales College of Medicine, 2002.

2 Farrell C, ed. *Patient and public involvement in health: The evidence for policy implementation. A summary of the results of the Health in Partnership research programme.* London: Department of Health Publications, April 2004. Available from: www.dh.gov.uk/en/Publicationsandstatistics/Publications/PublicationsPolicyAndGuidance/DH_4082332.

3 Adapted from Marshall T. Prevention of cardiovascular disease. Risk and benefit calculator. Available from: www.haps.bham.ac.uk/publichealth/cardiovascular/index.shtml.

4 Evans I, Thornton H. Transparency in numbers: the dangers of statistical illiteracy. *Journal of the Royal Society of Medicine* 2009;102:354-6.

5 Irwig L, Irwig J, Trevena L, *et al. Smart health choices: making sense of health advice.* London: Hammersmith Press, 2008.

6 Salzburg Global Seminar website: www.salzburgglobal.org.

7 Salzburg statement on shared decision making: Salzburg Global Seminar. *BMJ* 2011;342:d1745. Available from: www.bmj.com/content/342/bmj.d1745.full.

Chapter 13. Research for the right reasons: blueprint for a better future

1 Chalmers 1, Glasziou P. Avoidable waste in the production and reporting of research evidence. *Lancet* 2009;374:86-89.

2 Roberts I, Yates D, Sandercock P, *et al*; CRASH trial collaborators. Effect of intravenous corticosteroids on death within 14 days in 10008 adults with clinically significant head injury (MRC CRASH trial): randomised placebo-controlled trial. *Lancet* 2004;364:1321-8.

3 Cochrane Injuries Group Albumin Reviewers. Human albumin administration in critically ill patients: systematic review of randomised controlled trials. *BMJ* 1998;317:235-40.

4 Finfer S, Bellomo R, Bryce N, *et al* (SAFE Study Investigators). A comparison of albumin and saline for fluid resuscitation in the intensive care unit. *New England Journal of Medicine* 2004;350:2247-56.

5 Edwards A, Elwyn G, Atwell C, *et al.* Shared decision making and risk communication in general practice – a study incorporating systematic literature reviews, psychometric evaluation of outcome measures, and quantitative, qualitative and health economic analyses of a cluster randomised trial of professional skill development. Report to Health in Partnership programme, UK Department of Health. Cardiff: Department of General Practice. University of Wales College of Medicine, 2002.

6 Farrell C, ed. *Patient and public involvement in health: The evidence for policy implementation. A summary of the results of the Health in Partnership research programme.* London: Department of Health Publications, April 2004. Available from: www.dh.gov.uk/en/Publicationsandstatistics/Publications/PublicationsPolicyAndGuidance/DH_4082332.

7 Donovan J, Mills N, Smith M, *et al* for the ProtecT Study Group. Quality improvement report: improving design and conduct of randomised trials by embedding them in qualitative research: ProtecT (prostate testing for cancer and treatment) study. *BMJ* 2002;325:766-70.

8 Dickersin K, Chalmers I. Recognising, investigating and dealing with incomplete and biased reporting of clinical research: from Francis Bacon to the World Health Organization. James Lind Library, 2010 (www.jameslindlibrary.org).

9 Chan A-W, Hróbjartsson A, Haahr MT, *et al.* Empirical evidence for selective reporting of outcomes in randomized trials: comparison of protocols to published articles. *JAMA* 2004;291:2457-65.

10 Chan AW, Altman DG. Epidemiology and reporting of randomised trials published in PubMed journals. *Lancet* 2005;365:1159-62.

11 Glasziou P, Meats E, Heneghan C, Shepperd S. What is missing from descriptions of treatment in trials and reviews? *BMJ* 2008;336:1472-4.

12 Clarke M, Hopewell S, Chalmers I. Clinical trials should begin and end with systematic reviews of relevant evidence: 12 years and waiting. *Lancet* 2010;376:20-21.

Additional resources

DO YOU WANT FURTHER GENERAL INFORMATION ABOUT
TESTING TREATMENTS?

Websites

Testing Treatments Interactive
www.testingtreatments.org is where you will find a free electronic
version of the second edition of *Testing Treatments*, and where
translations and other material will be added over the coming years.
Translations of the first edition of *Testing Treatments* are available at
the site in Arabic, Chinese, German, Italian, Polish and Spanish.

James Lind Library
www.jameslindlibrary.org

Cochrane Collaboration
www.cochrane.org

NHS Choices
www.nhs.uk (enter 'research' in search window)

UK Clinical Research Collaboration
www.ukcrc.org

Healthtalkonline
www.healthtalkonline.org

US National Cancer Institute
Educational material about clinical trials
http://cancertrials.nci.nih.gov/clinicaltrials/learning

Books

Ben Goldacre. *Bad science*. London: Harper Perennial, 2009.

Bengt D Furberg, Curt D Furberg. *Evaluating clinical research: all that glitters is not gold*. 2nd edition. New York: Springer, 2007.

Steven Woloshin, Lisa Schwartz, Gilbert Welch. *Know your chances: understanding health statistics*. Berkeley: University of California Press, 2008. Available free at www.jameslindlibrary.org.

Les Irwig, Judy Irwig, Lyndal Trevena, Melissa Sweet. *Smart health choices: making sense of health advice*. London: Hammersmith Press, 2008. Available free at www.jameslindlibrary.org.

Trish Greenhalgh. *How to read a paper: the basics of evidence-based medicine.* 4th edition. Oxford and London: Wiley-Blackwell and BMJI Books, 2010.

H Gilbert Welch, Lisa M. Schwartz, Steven Woloshin. *Overdiagnosed: making people sick in the pursuit of health.* Boston: Beacon Press, 2011.

DO YOU WANT INFORMATION ABOUT WHAT IS KNOWN ABOUT THE EFFECTS OF TREATMENTS?

Cochrane Library
www.thecochranelibrary.com

NHS Evidence
www.evidence.nhs.uk

Informed Health Online
www.informedhealthonline.org

PubMed Health
www.pubmed.gov/health

DO YOU WANT INFORMATION ABOUT WHAT ISN'T KNOWN ABOUT THE EFFECTS OF TREATMENTS?

UK Database of Uncertainties about the Effects of Treatments (UK DUETs) www.evidence.nhs.uk

DO YOU WANT INFORMATION ABOUT CURRENT RESEARCH ADDRESSING UNCERTAINTIES ABOUT THE EFFECTS OF TREATMENTS?

WHO International Clinical Trials Registry Platform
www.who.int/trialsearch

US National Institutes of Health Clinical Trials Registry
www.clinicaltrials.gov

EU Clinical Trials Register
https://www.clinicaltrialsregister.eu

Australian Cancer Trials
www.australiancancertrials.gov.au

DO YOU WANT TO BECOME INVOLVED IN IMPROVING THE RELEVANCE AND QUALITY OF RESEARCH ON THE EFFECTS OF TREATMENTS?

James Lind Alliance
www.lindalliance.org
Promotes working partnerships between patients and clinicians to identify and prioritize important uncertainties about the effects of treatments.

National Institute for Health Research
NIHR Health Technology Assessment
www.ncchta.org
Actively involves service-users in all stages of its work.

NIHR Clinical Research Network Coordinating Centre
www.crncc.nihr.ac.uk/ppi
Keen to involve patients, carers, and the public in volunteering for clinical studies and getting actively involved as researchers.

Cochrane Consumer Network
www.consumers.cochrane.org
Promotes patient input to systematic reviews of treatments prepared by the Cochrane Collaboration.

UK Clinical Research Network
www.ukcrn.org.uk

DO YOU WANT TRAINING IN ASSESSING RESEARCH?

Critical Appraisal Skills Programme
www.casp-uk.net
Organizes workshops and other resources to help individuals to develop the skills to find and make sense of research evidence.

US Cochrane Center
Understanding Evidence-based Healthcare: A Foundation for Action
http://us.cochrane.org/understanding-evidence-based-healthcare-foundation-action
A web course designed to help individuals understand the fundamentals of evidence-based healthcare concepts and skills.

DO YOU WANT TO KNOW MORE ABOUT SHARED DECISION-MAKING?

The Foundation for Informed Medical Decision Making
www.informedmedicaldecisions.org
Dartmouth-Hitchcock Medical Center:
Center for Shared Decision Making
http://patients.dartmouth-hitchcock.org/shared_decision_making.html
Salzburg Statement
www.bmj.com/content/342/bmj.d1745.full
www.salzburgglobal.org

DO YOU WANT TO LEARN ABOUT SYSTEMATIC REVIEWS OF ANIMAL RESEARCH?

www.sabre.org.uk
www.camarades.info

List of Vignettes

Inquiry 2010;7(1):13-29. Available online: http://tinyurl.com/Spielmans.

p 100 **Science is cumulative but scientists don't accumulate evidence scientifically**
Goldacre B. Bad Science: How pools of blood trials could save lives. *The Guardian*, 10 May 2008, p16.

p 102 **Could checking the evidence first have prevented a death?**
Perkins E. Johns Hopkins Tragedy. *Information Today* 2001;18:51-54.

p 103 **Instructions to authors to put research results in context by the editors of the medical journal *The Lancet***
Clark S, Horton R. Putting research in context – revisited. *Lancet* 2010;376:10-11.

9. Regulating tests of treatments: help or hindrance?

p 105 **Who says medical research is bad for your health?**
Hope T. *Medical ethics: a very short introduction*. Oxford: Oxford University Press, 2004, p99.

p 108 **In an ideal world**
Goldacre B. Pharmaco-epidemiology would be fascinating enough even if society didn't manage it really really badly. *The Guardian*, 17 July 2010. Available online: www.badscience.net/2010/07/pharmaco-epidemiology-would-be-fascinating-enough-even-if-society-didnt-manage-it-really-really-badly.

p 109 **Biased ethics**
Lantos J. Ethical issues – how can we distinguish clinical research from innovative therapy?
American Journal of Pediatric Hematology/Oncology 1994; 16: 72-75.

p 110 **Rethinking informed consent**
Manson NC, O'Neill O. *Rethinking informed consent in bioethics*. Cambridge: Cambridge University Press, 2007, p200.

p 111 **A commonsense approach to informed consent in good medical practice**
Gill R. How to seek consent and gain understanding. *BMJ* 2010;341:c4000.

p 113 **Academic nicety – or sensible choice?**
Harrison J. Testing times for clinical research. *Lancet* 2006; 368:909-910.

p 114 **What research regulation should do**
Ashcroft, R. Giving medicine a fair trial. *BMJ* 2000;320:1686.

10. Research – good, bad, and unnecessary

p 117 **My experience of Magpie**
MRC News Release. Magnesium sulphate halves risk of eclampsia and can save lives of pregnant women. London: MRC, 31 May 2002.

p 124 **Impact of 'me-too' drugs in Canada**
Morgan SG, Bassett KL, Wright JM, *et al*. 'Breakthrough' drugs and growth in expenditure on prescription drugs in Canada. *BMJ* 2005;331:815-6.

List of Key Points

1. New – but is it better?

- Testing new treatments is necessary because new treatments are as likely to be worse as they are to be better than existing treatments
- Biased (unfair) tests of treatments can lead to patients suffering and dying
- The fact that a treatment has been licensed doesn't ensure that it is safe
- Side-effects of treatments often take time to appear
- Beneficial effects of treatments are often overplayed, and harmful effects downplayed

2. Hoped-for effects that don't materialize

- Neither theory nor professional opinion is a reliable guide to safe, effective treatments
- Just because a treatment is 'established' does not mean it does more good than harm
- Even if patients do not suffer from inadequately tested treatments, using them can waste individual and community resources

3. More is not necessarily better

- More intensive treatment is not necessarily beneficial, and can sometimes do more harm than good

4. Earlier is not necessarily better

- Earlier diagnosis does not necessarily lead to better outcomes; sometimes it makes matters worse
- Screening programmes should only be introduced on the basis of sound evidence about their effects
- Not introducing a screening programme can be the best choice
- People invited for screening need balanced information
- The benefits of screening are often oversold
- The harms of screening are often downplayed or ignored
- Good communication about the benefits, harms, and risks of screening is essential

5. Dealing with uncertainty about the effects of treatments

- Dramatic effects of treatments are rare
- Uncertainties about the effects of treatments are very common
- Small differences in the effects of different treatments are usual, and it is important to detect these reliably
- When nobody knows the answer to an important uncertainty about the effects of a treatment, steps need to be taken to reduce the uncertainty
- Much more could be done to help patients contribute to reducing uncertainties about the effects of treatments

6. Fair tests of treatment

- Fair tests of treatments are needed because we will otherwise sometimes conclude that treatments are useful when they are not, and vice versa
- Comparisons are fundamental to all fair tests of treatments
- When treatments are compared (or a treatment is compared with no treatment) the principle of comparing 'like with like' is essential
- Attempts must be made to limit bias in assessing treatment outcomes

7. Taking account of the play of chance

- Account must be taken of 'the play of chance' by assessing the confidence that can be placed in the quality and quantity of evidence available

8. Assessing all the relevant, reliable evidence

- A single study rarely provides enough evidence to guide treatment choices in healthcare
- Assessments of the relative merits of alternative treatments should be based on systematic reviews of all the relevant, reliable evidence
- As in individual studies testing treatments, steps must be taken to reduce the misleading influences of biases and the play of chance
- Failure to take account of the findings of systematic reviews has resulted in avoidable harm to patients, and wasted resources in healthcare and research

9. Regulating tests of treatments: help or hindrance?

- Regulation of research is unnecessarily complex
- Current systems of research regulation discourage fair tests of treatments that would make for better healthcare
- Despite the onerous regulatory requirements placed on researchers, regulatory systems do little to ensure that proposed studies are genuinely needed
- Research regulation does little to monitor and follow-up approved research

10. Research – good, bad, and unnecessary

- Unnecessary research is a waste of time, effort, money, and other resources; it is also unethical and potentially harmful to patients
- New research should only proceed if an up-to-date review of earlier research shows that it is necessary, and after it has been registered
- Evidence from new research should be used to update the previous review of all the relevant evidence
- Much research is of poor quality and done for questionable reasons
- There are perverse influences on the research agenda, from both industry and academia
- Questions that matter to patients are often not addressed

11. Getting the right research done is everybody's business

- Patients and researchers working together can help to identify and reduce treatment uncertainties
- Input from patients can lead to better research
- Patients sometimes inadvertently jeopardize fair tests of treatments
- Relationships between patients' organizations and the pharmaceutical industry can result in distorted information about treatment effects
- To contribute effectively, patients need better general knowledge about research and readier access to impartial information
- There is no one 'right way' of achieving collaborative participation in research
- Patient participation should be appropriate for the specific research purpose
- Methods of involving patients are continually evolving

Index

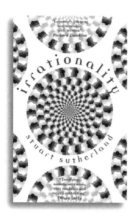
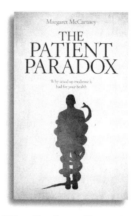
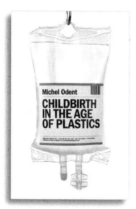
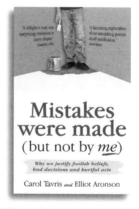